Dementia:

A Daughter's Journey to Prevention

by

Sandra Carol Pye

TABLE OF CONTENTS

ABOUT THE AUTHOR

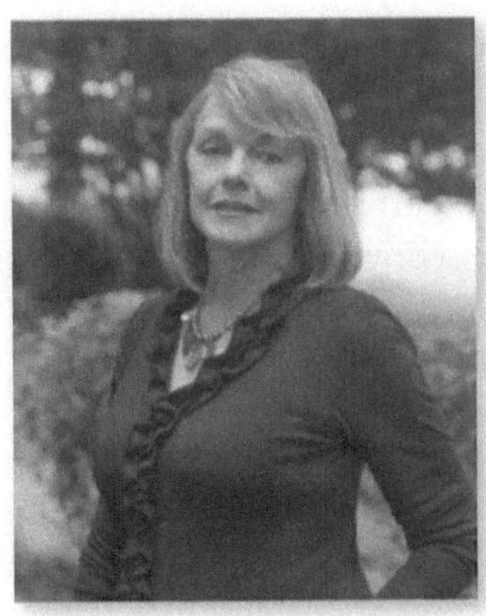

Sandra Carol Pye loves talking about happy childhood memories growing up on the family farm in Pinehurst, GA. As a high school student in Vienna, GA, the author developed a love of writing. Sandra loved working on short story and essay homework assignments. Many times she wrote while sitting on the creek bank listening to the peaceful sounds of nature.

After high school, Sandra studied Business Administration and Accounting at South GA Tech, Americus, GA. For a total of 33 years she worked for the State of Georgia at Georgia Southern University, University of Georgia, and the State Department of Education.

Sandra also studied Real Estate at Georgia Southern University and spent four years working as a real estate agent at Coldwell Banker Tanner Realty, Statesboro.

Sandra retired on December 31, 2006, two years earlier than planned when her Mother was in the mild stage of dementia.

By retiring earlier, Sandra could spend quality time with her Mother while she was still alert and able to walk with occasional assistance. They enjoyed trips to Tybee Island and Jekyll Island; this special time was spent walking barefoot on the sandy beaches,

http://SandraPye.com/contact

shopping, eating lots of great food, and just being together. Also, there were a couple of trips to the mountains shared with siblings that were a real treat for all with lots of fun and laughter. In the words of the author, it was *a wonderful and grand adventure.*"

Sandra's long-lost love of writing resurfaced after she retired. She enrolled in American Writers and Artists, Inc. (AWAI's) online writing classes and completed the education and training for the AWAI Program in Web Copywriting. With her book completed, Sandra will continue her freelance copywriting business at SandraPye.com and specialize in spreading the word about Dementia Prevention and Brain Health.

The author and her husband Joseph (Jr.) live in Statesboro, GA 75 miles west of Tybee Island, GA. They have a son Tim Pye, and a daughter Tammy Olliff. They are blessed to have Tim and Tammy and their families who also live in Statesboro.

DEDICATION

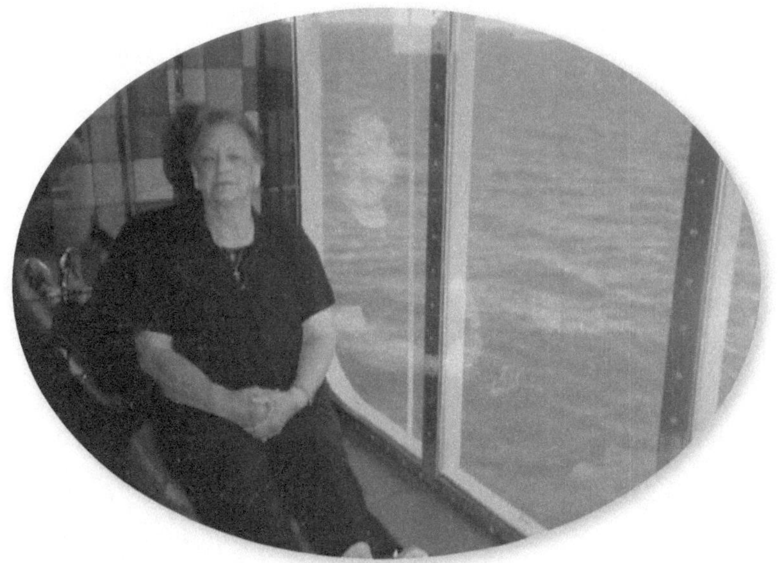

*In loving memory of Laura Inez Langford,
our sweet and beautiful Mother.*

*Photo taken during her six-day cruise to the Caribbean Islands
before dementia; a happy time in her life.*

ACKNOWLEDGMENTS

Heartfelt gratitude goes to my three siblings who also traveled this journey with mother-Margie, Covie, and Felicia. You lived closer to mother and took turns checking on her, took her to doctors' appointments, shopping, kept her checkbook in order, took her home cooked meals, and more. I appreciate everything you did and for "being there" for her when I couldn't. Thank you for your love and devotion to Mother, especially during her dementia illness. I love you all.

Many thanks to my loving husband Joseph (Jr.), son Tim, and daughter Tammy for encouraging me. Though you were surprised to learn that I was writing this book, you made no negative comments to discourage me and allowed me space and time without asking a million questions. You knew writing this book would be an emotional journey because I needed to draw from real life observations, experiences, some regrets, and select what I shared about Mother's illness. Mother's dignity and memory remained top priority as I wrote the book. Thank you for standing by me, I love you.

Thank you to our grandchildren: April, Morgan, Erin, and TJ for your encouragement (and also, the great grands: Keith, Holli and JT). Your kind and generous big hugs 'just because' were huge stress relievers for me (and still are!). Thank you to April for creating the colorful Dementia Umbrella artwork used in Chapter 1.

Thanks to Art Remnet at TheStrategicMarketingGroup.com whom I met through a Facebook copywriters' group. Art led a

Mastermind group and supported and encouraged the efforts for this book. I could not have done this without his suggestions, encouragement, and expertise in technology. Art's interest, along with experience and knowledge gained through being his Dad's caregiver during his dementia illness, became a common interest and concern about dementia prevention. Thank you Art.

A special thanks to Eileen Caswell, Editor at CaswellCopy.com. I am thankful for the opportunity to work with Eileen and form a special bond as we worked together to make this book a reality. Eileen was a joy to work with. As I waded into the unknown territory of writing a book and needed a top-notch editor, I found that Eileen was "the one" for my project. Eileen showed much interest in my topic throughout and added other interesting information she found along the way. Thank you, Eileen, for your time and dedication to this project.

This book would not be complete without the aid of Mary T. Newport, MD, a practicing Neonatologist for 29 plus years. Dr. Newport allowed me to share husband Steve's story about his battle with Alzheimer's disease. Diagnosed with Alzheimer's disease at age 53, Steve was sick for many years, and Dr. Newport continued to work much of the time. She was his primary caregiver during his illness through an incredible journey of research and discovering that the Medium Chain Triglycerides (MCT) Oil in Coconut Oil could help restore Steve's memory when taken daily.

Thank you for your generous input and invaluable information, for continuing your research, and for sharing the books you have written in memory of Steve.

You can read Steve's Story and find other book titles by Dr. Mary T. Newport in Chapter 7, Coconut Oil and MCT Oil.

Coconut Oil: Dietary Guidelines and Suggestions are located in the Appendix Section. *Report published with permission from Dr. Mary T. Newport, MD.*

For more information visit Dr. Mary Newport's website and blog:

- Coconutketones.com
- Coconutketones.blogspot.com

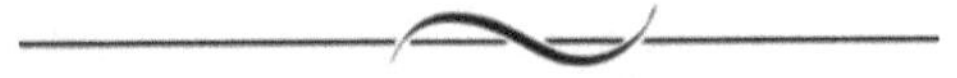

I am indebted to my dear mother, Laura Inez Langford.
I could not have written this book without
your love and strength to guide me.
I felt your sweet presence all around me.
You were a significant role model
who taught me honesty, strength, perseverance, and love.
I love you Mother and miss you and Dad always.

INTRODUCTION

A Mother's Love and Devotion

Growing up, Mother worked hard to take care of my brother, two sisters and me. She got up at 5:00 am Monday through Friday to cook breakfast for us before the school bus came. She then carpooled to and from work, a 30-minute trip each way. If Dad didn't have dinner cooked when she got home at 6:00 pm, Mother jumped in and cooked dinner for all of us.

To save money, Mother spent many hours after dinner sewing garments for us girls. I recall many nights getting up to find her still at the sewing machine at 1:00 am. determined to finish a skirt or a blouse for one of us to wear to school the next morning. I remember her coming home talking about her supervisor catching her dozing on the job and how hard it was to stay awake.

As an adult, I recognize the sacrifices that Mother made for us. As a role model, she taught us the value of hard work, perseverance, and family. However tired Mother may have been, she was always kind, loving and patient.

Looking back, I recognize that lack of sleep may have put Mother in the path of dementia and Alzheimer's.

I Continued to Be in Denial

We first noticed Mother having mild memory problems in early 2004 but attributed it to her age. Mother still lived in her own home and took care of herself. My brother and sister lived close by if she needed anything.

Summer of 2007, Mother's issues became more noticeable. As her illness progressed, I continued to deny what was happening. For every troubling sign of possible dementia, I observed, I believed the symptoms resulted from another illness. I was determined to find a problem that could be fixed.

Researching Other Illnesses that Could Mimic Dementia

Because I wanted to understand what mother was going through so that I could comfort and help her, I focused on researching illnesses that mimicked dementia.

The other possibility that I researched was if any of her medications she was taking could be causing the memory loss and confusion.

On several occasions, we expressed our concerns with Mother's doctor about her memory loss and disorientation. Each time he followed through by having her tested and reviewing her medications. Mother was admitted to the hospital several times; once to check her thyroid, once to check the carotid arteries, and once to check the hippocampus in the brain. The results of every test taken came back negative.

We hoped that Mother had another illness that could be 'fixed'.

Searching for a Solution to Bring our Beautiful Mother Back to Us

My siblings and I worked together throughout this sad journey to find an illness to *fix* that would bring Mother back to us. The fear and hopelessness she felt as she tried to form words and couldn't must have been profound. Instead, a garbled mix of words resulting in a partial sentence came out.

Frustrated, she stopped mid-sentence knowing she wasn't saying what she wanted. We tried to comfort her and calm her fears. We told her that the confusion may have been a side effect of a new medication she was taking.

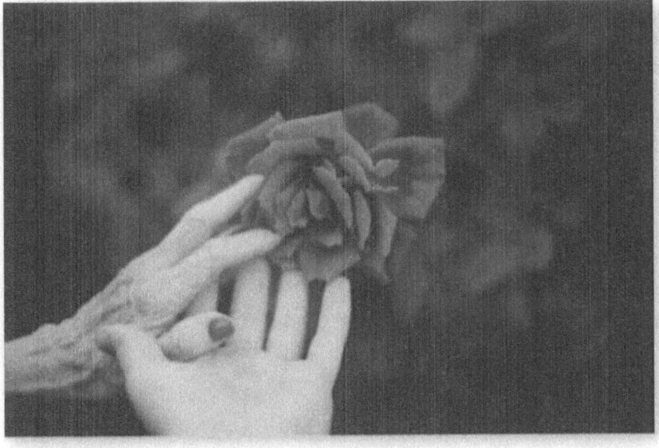

One night after Mother's disorientation and memory loss worsened, she had a bad fall. She hit her head and had to go to the emergency room for treatment. After the fall, she got progressively worse, and her doctor recommended we call hospice care. Soon after, she stopped trying to speak; eventually she no longer recognized her own children and grandchildren.

http://SandraPye.com/contact

To make a long, sad story short, the most painful time we fought to avoid had arrived. Our beautiful, once vibrant and happy Mother, had no more emotions or memories to share with us. She had been lost to dementia. Over the next few weeks, we continued to talk to Mother and gave her lots of hugs even though she could not communicate with us.

Mother passed away on December 26, 2008, the morning after our last Christmas day with her.

Painful Experience Left Me with a Sad and Bitter Heart

Not ready to say goodbye, I had not prepared my heart and soul for losing my mother. Guilty thoughts flooded my mind. Did I do enough early on when she experienced memory loss? I assumed they were *age-related* and *normal* 'senior moments.' Did I drive the four and a half-hour round trip often enough to help with her care and keep her active? Probably not.

I enjoyed camping out in the hospital room and stayed until she was released each time. Mother didn't care for being alone in the hospital at night. There were many times that I brought her to my home in Statesboro for two or three-week visits. However, after two weeks, she got homesick.

I Never Understood Dementia and had No Reason to Learn about It

I regret that I didn't make myself more aware of Mother's illness and research ways to improve her health with non-medical options. A diet with super brain foods, regular physical exercise, and mental activities could have moved her in a positive 'healthy brain' direction. Her memory loss and disorientation may have improved and prevented her downward spiral into the Mild Cognitive Impairment (MCI) stage and into dementia.

There Are Two Things that Have Given Me Peace

Mother knew she was loved as she watched her four children rally around her *searching for solutions* and having her tested for illnesses that mimicked dementia.

The second thing that gives us peace--we know Mother is in Heaven with the love of her life, our Dad.

To Avoid Going Down the Same Path

I continue to learn from this experience and do everything possible to avoid going down the same path that steals beautiful memories and thinking skills. Although this sad experience is hard to talk about, it drove me to find out all I can about dementia and what I need to do to keep my brain healthy and alert.

If only I had known then what I know now

I could have taken steps early on to help Mother reverse her occasional memory loss and disorientation.

Exercise, such as walking, and mental stimulation could have helped to build new brain cells.

Adding super brain foods to her diet, and helping her solve her sleep issues to get a good night's rest would have given Mother a fighting chance to reverse the dementia-like symptoms.

Deep in my heart I have an urgent need to share this experience and information with others and that is why I wrote this book.

I want to help you or a loved one prevent or reduce the risk of getting this dreadful disease and avoid this devastating journey.

There is plenty of information to learn about this disease, and the research continues. Take advantage of the research information in this book and take the steps necessary to improve your health. Continue learning how to keep your brain healthy and alert for the rest of your life.

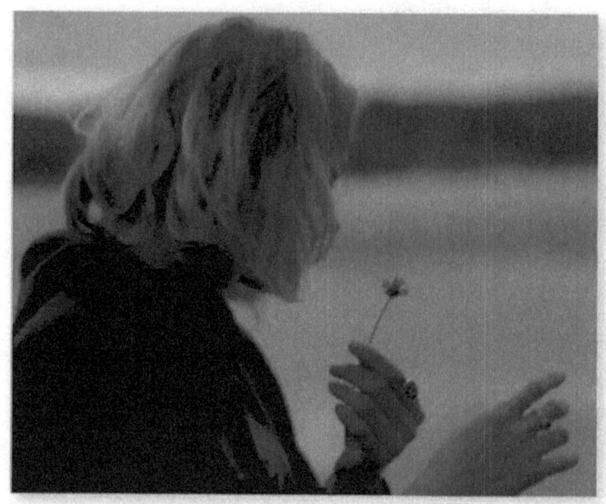

Looking back… reminiscing–remembering my happy, and not so happy memories.

Looking ahead…with determination to save ALL my memories that helped make me who I am and to keep making more sweet memories to cherish and remember for the rest of my life.

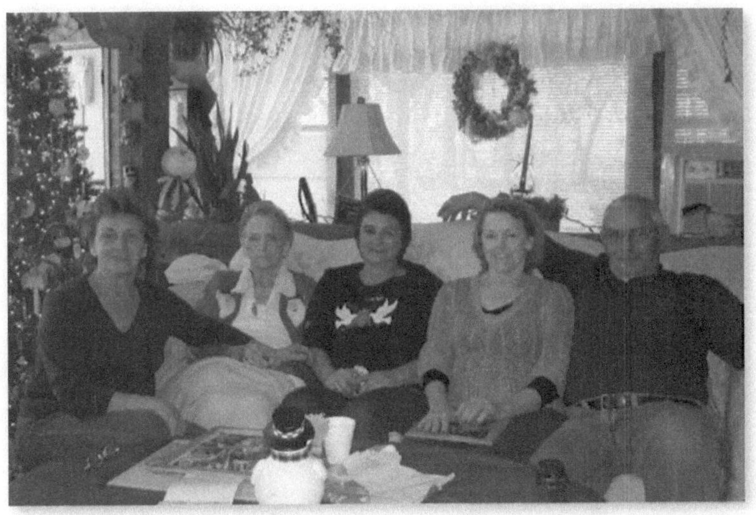

Mother dressed up for our 2008 family Christmas dinner with her children and grandchildren. We celebrated Christmas two weeks early to ensure she would be with us to celebrate. Unable to communicate or walk, Mother passed away the day after Christmas. (L-R: Sister – Margie Albritton, Mother, Sister – Felicia Harrell, me, and Brother – Covie Langford.)

SECTION 1:

"Under the Umbrella" of Dementia

CHAPTER 1

WHAT IS DEMENTIA AND WHAT ARE THE BROAD TYPES

Many would say that dementia is a group of thinking and social symptoms that interfere with daily functioning. But the truth is, the answer goes much deeper.

Dementia is not a specific disease. It's an overall term that describes a wide range of symptoms associated with a decline in memory or other thinking skills severe enough to reduce a person's ability to perform everyday activities.

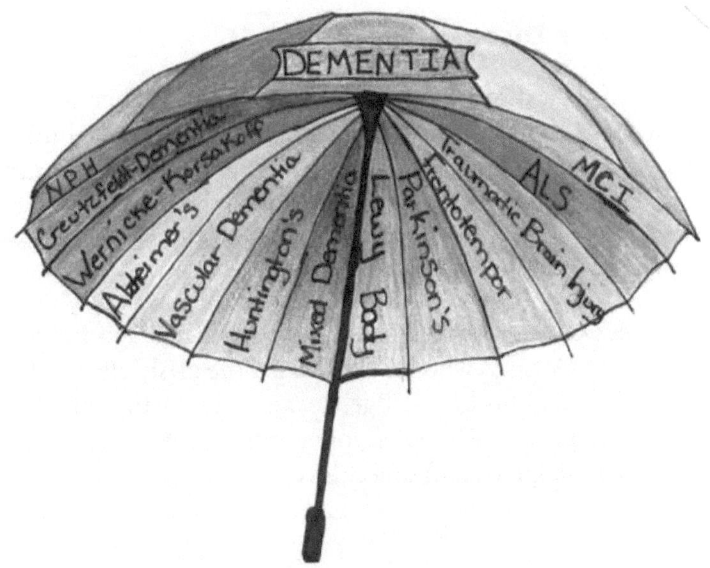

http://SandraPye.com/contact

Alzheimer's disease accounts for 60 to 80% of cases. Vascular dementia, which occurs after a stroke, is the second most common dementia type. But there are many other conditions that can cause symptoms of dementia, including some that are reversible, such as thyroid problems and Vitamin deficiencies.

Dementia is often incorrectly referred to as *"senility"* or *"senile dementia,"* which reflects the formerly widespread but incorrect belief that serious mental decline is a normal part of aging.

Dementia is caused when the brain is damaged by diseases, such as Alzheimer's disease or a series of strokes. Dementia is an **umbrella** term. It describes the symptoms that occur when the brain is affected by certain diseases or conditions. There are many types of dementia. Some of the more common types are outlined below.

Alzheimer's Disease

Alzheimer's is a disease that attacks the brain. Alzheimer's is a type of dementia that causes problems with memory, thinking and behavior. Alzheimer's is the most common form of dementia, a general term for memory loss and other intellectual abilities serious enough to interfere with daily life. Alzheimer's disease accounts for 60 to 80% of dementia case.

Alzheimer's disease was named nearly 100 years ago for Alois Alzheimer, a German who first described the grisly effects of the disease. To gather his knowledge, he cut away the tops of several skulls from people who died of a mind-destroying malady, leaving them helpless, and speechless.

He was probably the first to see inside a diseased brain and view the signature features of Alzheimer's. Alzheimer's method of diagnosis after death remains the only way to be absolutely certain of the disease even today. [3]

Symptoms: Difficulty remembering recent conversations, names or events is often an early clinical symptom; apathy and depression are also early symptoms. Later symptoms include impaired communication, poor judgment, disorientation, confusion, behavior changes and difficulty speaking, swallowing and walking.

Revised criteria and guidelines for diagnosing Alzheimer's were published in 2011 recommending that Alzheimer's be considered a slowly progressive brain disease that begins well before symptoms emerge.

Brain changes: Hallmark abnormalities are deposits of the protein fragment beta-amyloid (plaques) and twisted strands of the protein tau (tangles) as well as evidence of nerve cell damage and death in the brain.

Alzheimer's is not a normal part of aging, although the greatest known risk factor is increasing age, and the majority of people with Alzheimer's are 65 and older.

But Alzheimer's is not just a disease of old age. Up to five percent of people with the disease have early onset Alzheimer's (also known as younger-onset), which often appears when someone is in their 40s or 50s.

Alzheimer's worsens over time. Alzheimer's is a progressive disease, where dementia symptoms gradually worsen over a number of years. In its early stages, memory loss is mild, but with late-stage Alzheimer's, individuals lose the ability to carry on a conversation and respond to their environment. Alzheimer's is the sixth leading cause of death in the United States. Those with Alzheimer's live an average of eight years after their symptoms become noticeable to others, but survival can range from four to 20 years, depending on age and other health conditions. The most common early symptom of Alzheimer's is difficulty remembering newly learned information because Alzheimer's changes typically begin in the part of the brain that affects learning.

As Alzheimer's advances through the brain it leads to increasingly severe symptoms, including disorientation, mood and behavior changes; deepening confusion about events, time and place; unfounded suspicions about family, friends and professional caregivers; more serious memory loss and behavior changes; and difficulty speaking, swallowing and walking.

Vascular Dementia

Previously known as multi-infarct or post-stroke dementia, vascular dementia is less common as a sole cause of dementia than Alzheimer's, accounting for about ten percent of dementia cases.

Symptoms: Impaired judgment or ability to make decisions, plan or organize is more likely to be initial symptoms, as opposed to the memory loss often associated with the initial symptoms of Alzheimer's. This disorder caused by blood vessel blockage or damage leads to infarcts (strokes) or bleeding in the brain. The location, number and size of the brain injury determine how the individual's thinking and physical functioning are affected.

Brain changes: Brain imaging can often detect blood vessel problems implicated in vascular dementia. In the past, evidence for vascular dementia was used to exclude a diagnosis of Alzheimer's disease (and vice versa). That practice is no longer considered consistent with pathologic evidence, which shows that the brain changes of several types of dementia can be present simultaneously. When any two or more types of dementia are present at the same time, the individual is considered to have "mixed dementia" (see entry below).

Dementia with Lewy Bodies (DLB)

Most experts estimate that dementia with Lewy bodies is the third most common cause of dementia after Alzheimer's disease and vascular dementia, accounting for 10 to 25% of cases.

Symptoms: People with dementia with Lewy bodies often have memory loss and thinking problems common in Alzheimer's, but are more likely than people with Alzheimer's to have initial or early symptoms such as sleep disturbances, well-formed visual hallucinations, and slowness, gait imbalance or other parkinsonian movement features.

Brain changes: Lewy bodies are abnormal aggregations (or clumps) of the protein alpha-synuclein. When they develop in a part of the brain called the cortex, dementia can result. Alpha-synuclein also aggregates in the brains of people with Parkinson's disease, but the aggregates may appear in a pattern that is different from dementia with Lewy bodies.

The brain changes of dementia with Lewy bodies alone can cause dementia, or they can be present at the same time as the brain changes of Alzheimer's disease and/or vascular dementia, with each abnormality contributing to the development of dementia. When this happens, the individual is said to have "mixed dementia."

Mixed Dementia

In mixed dementia abnormalities linked to more than one cause of dementia occur simultaneously in the brain. Recent studies suggest that mixed dementia is more common than previously thought.

Symptoms: Mixed dementia symptoms may vary, depending on the types of brain changes involved and the brain regions affected. In many cases, symptoms may be similar to or even indistinguishable from those of Alzheimer's or another type of dementia. In other cases, a person's symptoms may suggest that more than one type of dementia is present.

Brain changes: Characterized by the hallmark abnormalities of more than one cause of dementia —most commonly, Alzheimer's and vascular dementia, but also other types, such as dementia with Lewy bodies.

Parkinson's Disease

As Parkinson's disease progresses, it often results in a progressive dementia similar to dementia with Lewy bodies or Alzheimer's.

Symptoms: Problems with movement are common symptoms of the disease. If dementia develops, symptoms are often similar to dementia with Lewy bodies.

Brain changes: Alpha-synuclein clumps are likely to begin in an area deep in the brain called the substantia nigra. These clumps are thought to cause degeneration of the nerve cells that produce dopamine.

Frontotemporal Dementia Includes:

- Behavioral variant FTD (bvFTD),
- Primary progressive aphasia,
- Pick's disease,
- Corticobasal syndrome, and,
- Progressive supranuclear palsy.

Symptoms: Typical symptoms include changes in personality and behavior and difficulty with language. Nerve cells in the front and side regions of the brain are especially affected.

Brain changes: No distinguishing microscopic abnormality is linked to all cases. People with FTD generally develop symptoms at a younger age (at about age 60) and survive for fewer years than those with Alzheimer's.

Creutzfeldt - Jakob Disease

CJD is the most common human form of a group of rare, fatal brain disorders known as Prion Disease affecting people and certain other mammals. Variant CJD (mad cow disease) occurs in cattle, and has been transmitted to people under certain circumstances.

Symptoms: Rapidly fatal disorder that impairs memory and coordination and causes behavior changes.

Brain changes: Results from misfolded prion protein that causes a "domino effect" in which prion protein throughout the brain misfolds and thus malfunctions.

Normal Pressure Hydrocephalus

Normal pressure hydrocephalus occurs when excess cerebrospinal fluid accumulates in the brain's ventricles, which are hollow fluid-filled chambers. NPH is called "normal pressure" because despite the excess fluid, cerebrospinal fluid pressure as measured during a spinal tap is often normal. As brain ventricles enlarge with the excess cerebrospinal fluid, they can disrupt and damage nearby brain tissue, causing symptoms of NPH.

NPH primarily affects people in their 60s and 70s. Scientists aren't certain how many older adults have this disorder because common symptoms of NPH are also common in other brain disorders.

Symptoms:

Difficulty walking that's sometimes compared to the way a person walks "on a boat," with the body bent forward, legs held wide apart and feet moving as if they're "glued to the deck."

Decline in thinking skills that includes overall slowing of thought processes, apathy, impaired planning and decision-making, reduced concentration and changes in personality and behavior.

Loss of bladder control, which tends to appear somewhat later in the disease than difficulty walking and cognitive decline.

Brain changes: Caused by the buildup of fluid in the brain, can sometimes be corrected with surgical installation of a shunt **in the brain** to drain excess fluid.

Huntington's Disease

Huntington's disease is a progressive brain disorder caused by a single defective gene on chromosome 4 – one of the 23 human chromosomes that carry a person's entire genetic code.

Symptoms: Include abnormal involuntary movements, a severe decline in thinking and reasoning skills, including memory, concentration, judgment and ability to plan and organize.

Brain changes: The gene defect causes abnormalities in a brain protein that, over time, lead to worsening symptoms.

Changes lead to alterations in mood, especially depression, anxiety, and uncharacteristic anger and irritability. Another common symptom is obsessive-compulsive behavior, leading a person to repeat the same question or activity over and over.

Wernicke-Korsakoff Syndrome

Wernicke-Korsakoff Syndrome is a chronic memory disorder caused by severe deficiency of thiamine (Vitamin B-1). The most common cause is alcohol misuse.

Symptoms: Memory problems may be strikingly severe while other thinking and social skills seem relatively unaffected.

Brain changes: Thiamine helps brain cells produce energy from sugar. When thiamine levels fall too low, brain cells cannot generate enough energy to function properly.

Traumatic Brain Injury (TBI)

Traumatic brain injury results from an impact to the head that disrupts normal brain function. Traumatic brain injury may affect a person's cognitive abilities, including learning and thinking skills. Falls are the leading cause of traumatic brain injury for all ages. Those aged 75 and older have the highest rates of traumatic brain injury-related hospitalization and death due to falls.

Doctors classify traumatic brain injury as mild, moderate or severe, depending on whether the injury causes unconsciousness, how long unconsciousness lasts and the severity of symptoms. Although most traumatic brain injuries are classified as mild because they're not life-threatening, even a mild traumatic brain injury can have serious and long-lasting effects. The severity of symptoms depends on whether the injury is mild, moderate or severe.

Symptoms:

- Unconsciousness
- Inability to remember the cause of the injury or events that occurred immediately before or up to 24 hours after
- Confusion and disorientation
- Difficulty remembering new information
- Headache
- Dizziness
- Blurry vision
- Nausea and vomiting
- Ringing in the ears
- Trouble speaking coherently
- Changes in emotions or sleep patterns

Brain Changes: Traumatic brain injury is a threat to cognitive health in two ways:

1. A traumatic brain injury's direct effects, which may be long-lasting or even permanent, can include unconsciousness, inability to recall the traumatic event, confusion, difficulty learning and remembering new information, trouble speaking coherently, unsteadiness, lack of coordination and problems with vision or hearing.

2. Certain types of traumatic brain injury may increase the risk of developing Alzheimer's or another form of dementia years after the injury takes place.

Mild Cognitive Impairment

Mild Cognitive Impairment (MCI) causes a slight but noticeable and measurable decline in cognitive abilities, including memory and thinking skills. A person with MCI is at an increased risk of developing Alzheimer's or another dementia.

Symptoms: Experts classify mild cognitive impairment based on the thinking skills affected:

- MCI that primarily affects memory is known as "amnestic MCI." With amnestic MCI, a person may start to forget important information that he or she would previously have recalled easily, such as appointments, conversations or recent events.
- MCI that affects thinking skills other than memory is known as "non-amnestic MCI." Thinking skills that may be affected by non-amnestic MCI include the ability to make sound decisions, judge the time or sequence of steps needed to complete a complex task, or visual perception.

Brain changes: Mild cognitive impairment causes cognitive changes that are serious enough to be noticed by the individuals experiencing them or to other people, but the changes are not severe enough to interfere with daily life or independent function.

Those with MCI have an increased risk of eventually developing Alzheimer's or another type of dementia. However, not all people with MCI get worse and some eventually get better. [1]

ALS (Amyotrophic Lateral Sclerosis) -- also known as Lou Gehrig's disease in the United States.

ALS is a disease of the parts of the nervous system that control voluntary muscle movement. In ALS, motor neurons (nerve cells that control muscle cells) are gradually lost. As these motor neurons are lost, the muscles they control become weak and then nonfunctional.

The word "amyotrophic" comes from Greek roots that mean "without nourishment to muscles" and refers to the loss of signals nerve cells normally send to muscle cells. "Lateral" means "to the side" and refers to the location of the damage in the spinal cord. "Sclerosis" means "hardened" and refers to the hardened nature of the spinal cord in advanced ALS.

In the United States, ALS also is called Lou Gehrig's disease, named after the Yankees baseball player who died of it in 1941. In the United Kingdom and some other parts of the world, ALS is often called *motor neuron* disease in reference to the cells that are lost in this disorder.

Symptoms: ALS results in muscles that are weak and soft, or stiff, tight and spastic. Muscle twitches and cramps are common; they occur because degenerating axons (long fibers extending from nerve-cell bodies) become "irritable."

Symptoms may be limited to a single body region, or mild symptoms may affect more than one region. When ALS begins in the bulbar motor neurons, the muscles used for swallowing and speaking are affected first. Rarely, symptoms begin in the respiratory muscles.

As ALS progresses, symptoms become more widespread, and some muscles become paralyzed while others are weakened or unaffected. In late-stage ALS, most voluntary muscles are paralyzed.

The involuntary muscles, such as those that control the heartbeat, gastrointestinal tract and bowel, bladder and sexual functions are not directly affected in ALS. Sensations, such as vision, hearing and touch, are also unaffected.

Brain changes: In most cases, ALS does not affect a person's thinking ability. However, some people with ALS develop some degree of cognitive (thinking) or behavioral abnormality. Usually, cognitive and behavioral symptoms in ALS range from mild (such that only close family members may notice a difference) to moderate. [2]

References:

1. Alzheimer's Association website
   http://www.alz.org/what-is-dementia.asp

2. Muscular Dystrophy Association
   https://www.mda.org/disease/amyotrophic-lateral-sclerosis

3. Losing My Mind – *An Intimate Look at Life with Alzheimer's by* Thomas DeBaggio. Copyright ©2002 – by Thomas DeBaggio. First Free Press Paperback Edition 2003

To learn more about Thomas DeBaggio visit:
https://en.wikipedia.org/wiki/Thomas_DeBaggio

SECTION II

Preventing Dementia "One Day At A Time"

CHAPTER 2

WHAT I DO TO PREVENT LOWER MY RISK FOR DEMENTIA

There are many things that you can do to prevent dementia. My plan to nurture and maintain a healthy brain is in place with add-ons from my ongoing research. I started to research information to create a simple *road map* to help me stay on track and accomplish my goal.

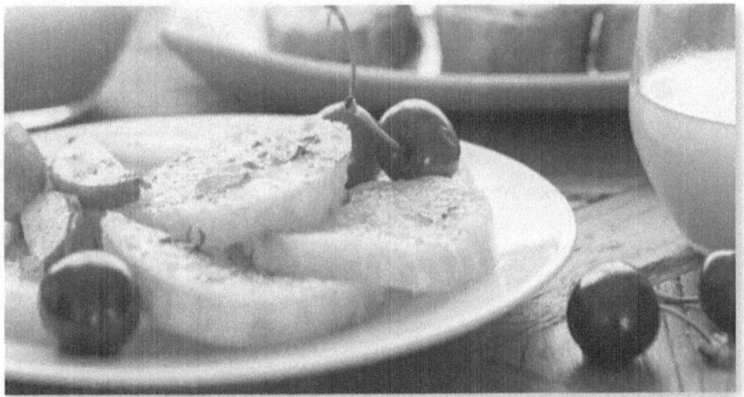

Along the way, I felt the need to share my experience to help others who want to save themselves or their loved ones from this devastating journey. By providing you quality information from reliable sources, you too, can create a plan that works for you.

http://SandraPye.com/contact

I Focused On Four Categories for This Book:

- DIETARY – Chapter 3,
- PHYSICAL ACTIVITIES – Chapter 4,
- MENTAL ACTIVITIES – Chapter 5, and
- WELLNESS – Chapter 6.

Under these four categories, I listed six items that the Alzheimer's Association recommends that you can do to help prevent dementia. In this chapter, I listed some of the steps I've *taken to prevent or reduce my risk of dementia* for reference. In Chapters 3-6, I broke these categories down further and listed the source of my research information. As you create your plan, be sure to include some of these recommendations or other suggestions that may work for you.

1. Eat Healthy.

2. Exercise regularly.

3. Be consistent with mental stimulation.

4. Get a good night's rest.

5. Stop smoking.

6. Keep blood pressure at a healthy level.

Eat Healthy

My favorite super brain foods are blueberries, strawberries, cranberries, tuna, trout, walnuts, broccoli, cabbage, kale, asparagus, red seedless grapes, and collard greens. My favorite drinks are green tea and my morning cup of coffee. *Coffee is not on the super brain list; but it's what I LOVE first thing every morning.*

I eat some of these foods every day and here's how I do it.

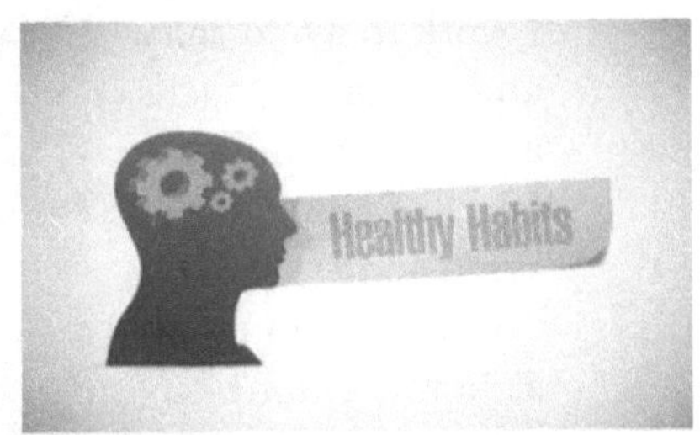

- Almost every morning for breakfast, I mix
  - 1½ ounces fresh blueberries or sliced strawberries and
  - 1½ ounces chopped walnuts with
  - 2½ ounces non-fat Greek yogurt-assorted flavors or plain.

Blueberries, strawberries, and walnuts are super brain foods and, when mixed with non-fat Greek yogurt, is very nutritious and delicious.

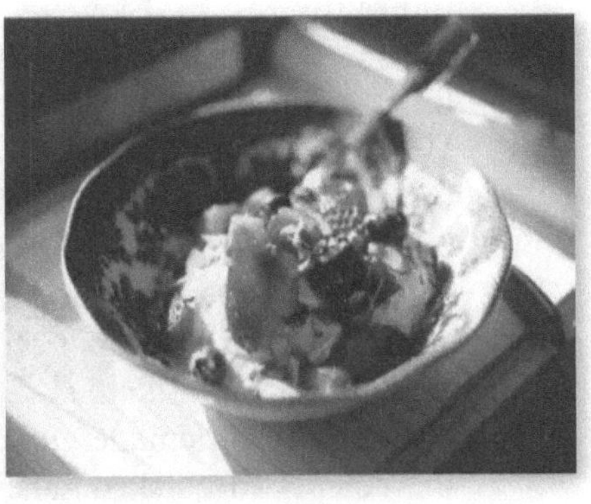

I prefer OIKOS yogurt (Triple Zero) in the 5.3 ounce round black carton with 15 grams of protein per carton and less sugar than others. This $1.00 size provides me two yogurt servings for two days with 7 1/2 grams of protein each morning.

This is a super healthy and delicious breakfast. If I miss this at breakfast, I will eat it for an afternoon snack and sometimes, stir in a small dollop of lite cool whip.

- I work to avoid salty and sugary snacks as much as possible and choose super brain-food snacks. To avoid temptation at home, I don't buy salty and sugary snacks anymore and prefer to eat fresh fruit super brain foods such as *strawberries and blueberries.* 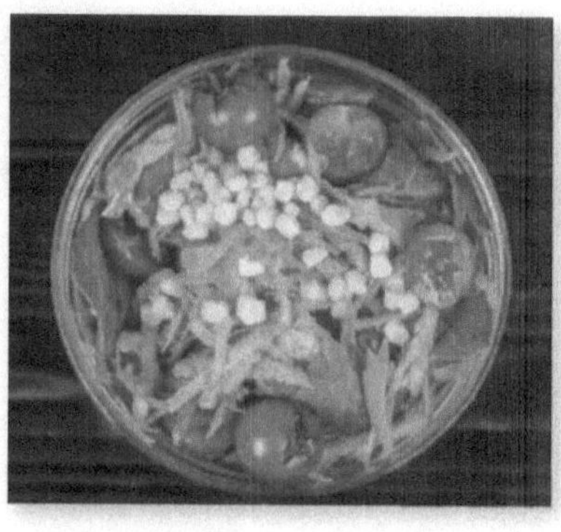

- Red seedless *grapes* are chilled to munch on in place of unhealthy snacks. I love *red grapes* and *walnuts* cut up in tuna salad and chicken salad for a healthy choice at lunch or dinner.

- With most meals, I eat a *green salad* with super brain foods such as *baby spinach* and *dried cranberries,* tossed in with grape tomatoes and cucumbers. For a twist, I will sometimes add carrots and corn to my salads.

- At least twice per week, I eat *fish.* My favorites are *tuna,* grilled *trout,* and *salmon.*

- I love my homemade *tuna* salad and add the same ingredients to chicken salad: diced 'bread and butter' pickles, halve or quarter *red* seedless *grapes,* add chopped *walnuts,* lite mayo, lite salt, and pepper.

- Homemade tuna or chicken salad makes delicious sandwiches with *100% whole wheat bread with 13 grams whole grain* for lunches. For convenience, I keep canned *tuna* on hand when I need to prepare a quick nutritious meal.

- During the day, I drink hot *green tea* if I need to relax or want to read. I drink green tea with ice and lemon with meals and keep a pitcher of green tea made with little sugar in the refrigerator.

- Each day I try to drink 6 six-ounce glasses of *water flavored with lemon.*

Brain foods are priority items on my grocery shopping list. I print copies to check off items I need at the grocery store.

Refer to Chapter 3, DIETARY, for more information about super brain foods and a sample of my **Shopping List with Super Brain Foods** *you can download and print.*

Exercise Regularly

Five miles from my home, there is a regional water park with a walking trail around the pond. This is a very tranquil place to walk. Studies show that physical activity such as walking is beneficial for your brain and body. I walk *at least* three days per week for 30 minutes, most of the time at this water park.

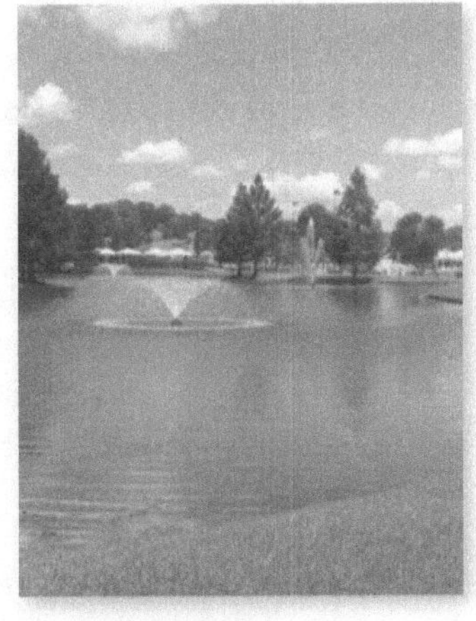

When I can't walk due to weather, I ride my stationary bike 30 minutes. This exercise keeps my blood flowing and helps ensure that my brain gets the blood and oxygen it needs to be healthy.

Learn more about the benefits of walking and other forms of exercise in Chapter 4, PHYSICAL ACTIVITIES.

Be Consistent with Mental Stimulation

Consistent mental exercise is critical to maintaining good brain health. I love reading and learning something interesting every day, and I find this to be an enjoyable way to stimulate my brain. I enjoy writing; this book has required a lot of daily mental stimulation. I enjoy researching the internet for answers to questions that come up daily. You may like to assemble jigsaw puzzles, work crossword, Sudoku, or word search puzzles to stretch your brain.

I have never watched much TV during the day. I try to stay active and encourage you to do the same.

Socialization is another method that can be used to stimulate the brain. I attend church and stay involved with church activities and interact with friends there. We discuss current topics, the weekly sermon, and catch up on what family members are doing.

During the week, I go out almost daily to run errands or meet a family member or friend for breakfast or lunch, and do personal shopping as needed. So, I am interacting with people I meet along the way; an important link to maintaining and strengthening a person's mental stamina.

The key is to find a favorite activity that you can enjoy doing daily to keep your mind stimulated and sharp!

Read Chapter 5 – MENTAL ACTIVITIES for more information and suggestions to help you choose daily activities that can strengthen your mental stamina.

Get a Good Night's Sleep

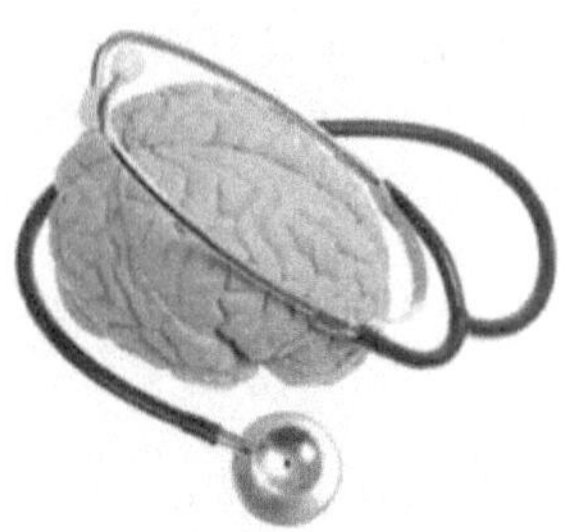

I try to get a good night's sleep every night, and my goal is eight hours. It is very important for me to get an adequate amount of sleep every night to feel rested the next day. This helps prevent achy muscles and to be able to think clearly all day. Adequate sleep is critical as I continue to manage Fibromyalgia.

Refer to Chapter 6, WELLNESS, for suggestions to help you work on improving your sleep routine each night.

Stop Smoking

I have never smoked except for the time I got caught trying to smoke a cigarette with a preacher's daughter at my house during seventh grade. Dad found out as we were about to get started and *invited me* to sit down at the table. He supervised *my* first smoking experience with half a cigarette. I coughed, spit and sputtered and had to put it down. I never wanted to smoke again. That was a thankful life lesson from my dad.

Refer to Chapter 6, WELLNESS, to learn more about the harmful effects smoking can have on your brain health.

Keep Blood Pressure at a Healthy Level

To reduce sodium intake, I use lite-salt (in the small, round, light blue container) sparingly when I cook. I also cook with coconut oil. If you do not like the taste of coconut, choose *refined,* or *all natural* or *RBD* (refined bleached, and deodorized). If you do like the taste of coconut, you may want to choose *virgin, organic,* or unrefined which are generally more expensive.

You can read more about this in-depth in Dr. Mary Newport's report later in this book.

I also gave up potato chips (even my favorite sour cream and cheddar chips). They are a reminder of raised blood pressure and other health problems; they are not worth the risk and are no longer a temptation. I regularly monitor my blood pressure at home. I will also check it if I have a headache since it is a symptom of HBP.

Refer to Chapter 6, WELLNESS, to learn more about the harmful effects of uncontrolled high blood pressure on the brain.

Take Coconut Oil Daily

I take one Tbsp of coconut oil in the morning and again in the evening. *You will learn more about Coconut Oil and its benefits in Chapter 7.*

Refer to Chapter 7 PROMISING RESEARCH-Coconut Oil and MCT Oil (Medium Chain Triglycerides) and learn How Coconut Oil with MCT Oil Feeds and Nurtures Your Brain

For more tips about adding coconut oil to your diet refer

The following information was found while learning about promising research to reverse memory loss and prevent or reduce the risk of dementia.

I added these two items to my personal to-do-list and think you will find them to be of great value.

The study, research, and clinical trials are ongoing and appear to hold much promise.

to *Chapter 7, Coconut Oil: Dietary Guidelines and Suggestions.*
Article published with permission from Dr. Mary T. Newport, MD.

NOTE: When selecting coconut oil, it is very important to choose
'*non-hydrogenated*' which contains no cholesterol or trans-fat.

Check Your Vitamin D Level

I take two 2000 IU Vitamin D3 supplements daily. My physician
recommended it to me based on blood work results after an
annual physical. I continue to do this for good brain health
maintenance.

Since then, I have learned that studies suggest a lack of Vitamin
D is linked to an increased risk of Alzheimer's disease. A study
published in 2014 by the Alzheimer's Society found people with
low Vitamin D levels were more than twice as likely to develop
some type of dementia. That got my attention!

*Refer to Chapter 9, PROMISING RESEARCH: Vitamin D
Deficiency Linked to Dementia, to learn how a deficiency can
affect your brain health.*

Photo Credits:

- Healthy Habits – Alexmillos - Canstockphoto.com
- Brain image – Homestudio - Canstockphoto.com

SECTION III

4 Areas of Emphasis to Prevent Dementia

CHAPTER 3

DIETARY

Eat Healthy

Can Eating More Fish and Walnuts Reduce My Risk of Dementia?

YES! You are probably thinking "why fish and walnuts"? Both are high in Omega-3 Fatty Acids and are excellent food sources to improve and maintain good brain health. The body doesn't produce fatty acids naturally and must be added. You can create a healthy and balanced diet eating foods rich in DHA Omega-3 Fatty Acids, Vitamins, and nutrients.

So let's talk about getting more DHA Omega-3 Fatty Acids in your diet. Fish and walnuts provide two foods high in Omega-3 Fatty Acids in order for you to receive the long-term benefits for your brain health. The expert on Omega-3 Fatty Acids is Dr. Frank Sacks at Harvard T.H. Chan School of Public Health.

Dr. Sacks states there are two major types of Omega-3 Fatty Acids in our diets:

- One type is alpha-linoleic acid (ALA), which is found in walnuts and some vegetable oils, such as soybean, rapeseed (canola), and flaxseed. ALA is also found in some green vegetables, such as Brussels sprouts, kale, spinach, and salad greens.

- The other type, eicosapentaenoic acid (EPA) and docosahexaenoic acid (DHA), is found in fatty fish.
- The body partially converts ALA to EPA and DHA.

It is not known whether vegetable or fish DHA Omega-3 Fatty Acids are equally beneficial, although both seem to be beneficial. For good health, you should aim to get at least one rich source of Omega-3 Fatty Acids in your diet every day. This could be through a serving of fatty fish such as salmon, or a handful of walnuts or ground flaxseed mixed into your morning oatmeal. [1]

PART I - Fish

Fatty fish—like salmon, mackerel, and herring— is the main source of docosahexaenoic acid (DHA), an omega-3 fatty acid key to brain health.

People who eat foods rich in DHA are nearly 40% less likely to develop Alzheimer's disease.

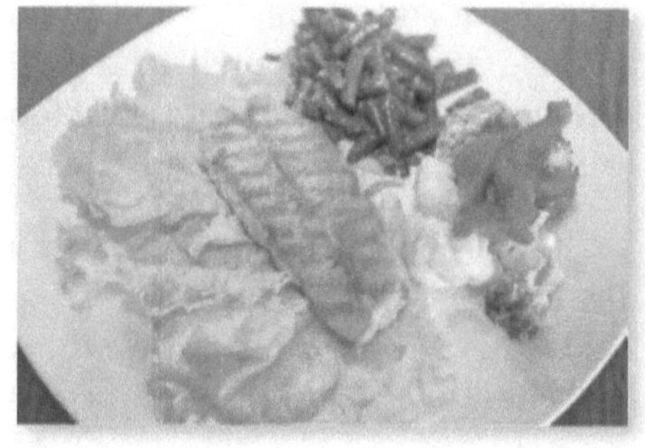

The results of a study on DHA levels by Tufts University researchers involved 899 men and women. Their average age was 76 and the average follow-up was just over nine years.

Their explanation of the results is as follows: People with the highest blood levels of DHA were 47% less likely to develop dementia of any kind, and 39% less likely to develop Alzheimer's compared to those with lower DHA levels.

Not surprisingly, people with the highest DHA levels also ate more fish. Three servings a week seems like the magic number.

Besides salmon, mackerel, and herring, good options include: tuna, shad, whitefish, trout, sardines, sablefish, bass, pompano, bluefish, oysters, halibut, and cod. [2]

PART II - Walnuts

Let's continue the discussion from Part 1 about getting more DHA Omega-3 Fatty Acids in your diet with walnuts, a food source high in Omega-3 Fatty Acids.

Have you ever thought about how the walnut and the human brain are shaped alike? Or have you noticed that the lines on the outside shell and on the nut resemble a human brain? It may be just a coincidence or a clear sign that this nut is a super brain food to eat and enjoy for brain health benefits.

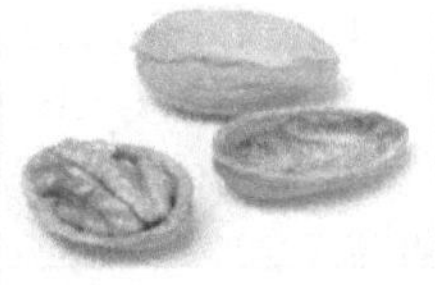
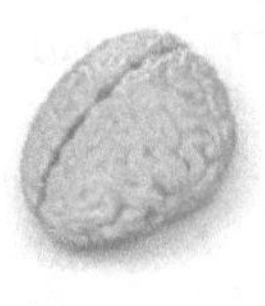

The walnut has achieved super brain food status due to brain-boosting properties known to fight Alzheimer's. The walnut is high in Omega-3 Fatty Acids, full of healthy fats, antioxidants, fiber, and lots of vitamins and minerals.

What are other benefits?

- Walnuts are high in Vitamin E, folate, and melatonin which improve cognitive skills.
- Walnuts are high in antioxidants which help inflammation and can also protect cells.
- Walnuts can also help the heart cope in times of stress.

Sometimes, simple foods are better for your health, as with walnuts. Eat just one 1.5 oz serving of walnuts daily and take advantage of their beneficial properties for good brain health.

Are you ready to boost your defense against dementia with fish and walnuts?

Strategy: Commit to eating more specific super brain foods daily such as fish and walnuts high in Omega-3 Fatty Acids to build new brain cells. It will help to prevent/reduce your risk of dementia as well as improve and maintain good brain health.

Suggestions for Fish:

- Add more fish to your diet and commit to eating at least two servings of fish each week.
- For variety, you can choose from: mackerel, herring, tuna, shad, whitefish, trout, sardines, sablefish, bass, pompano, bluefish, oysters, halibut, and cod.
- Here's a suggestion that I grew up with for breakfast, lunch, or dinner. Cook and scramble eggs and salmon together and serve over buttered grits. Another treat that I enjoyed was Mother's homemade biscuits filled with my grandmother's homemade pear preserves straight from our own pear tree. Those are happy memories too.

Suggestions for Walnuts:

- Grab a handful for a quick, on-the-go, nutritious snack. Prepare ahead and fill seven zip-lock snack bags with 1.5 – 2 oz for a week's supply and you have ready-to-go snacks. I add the super food, dried cranberries, to the bag for an added sweet treat.

- Add chopped walnuts to non-fat Greek yogurt, salads, tuna salad, chicken salad, and desserts.
- Create a master list of foods that contain Alpha-linoleic acid (ALA) and place in a binder. As you prepare your shopping list, be sure to include foods on the master list including vegetable oils, such as soybean, rapeseed (canola), and flaxseed. ALA is also found in some green vegetables, such as Brussels sprouts, kale, spinach, and salad greens.

To Prevent Memory Decline, Eat More Blueberries

BLUEBERRIES! Here is a fun food we can all enjoy all kinds of ways by folks of all ages from 2 to 102!

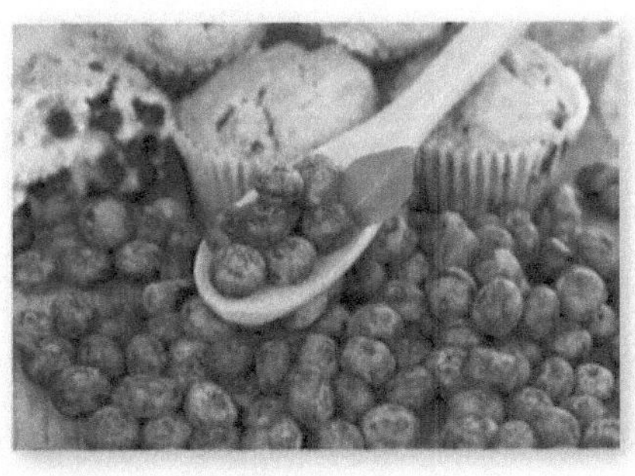

Blueberries are delicious and nutritious with only 80 calories per cup; they are an excellent source of food for good brain health.

Keep fresh and/or frozen blueberries on hand, and your family can have fun creating their blueberry treats with this versatile, low-fat, low-sodium fruit.

These tasty gems offer many nutritional benefits. They are rich in carotenoids and flavonoids and they are an excellent source of manganese.

Blueberries are packed with Vitamins C and K. They have enough dietary fiber to keep the body regular, the heart healthy, and cholesterol in check.

What's New and Beneficial About Blueberries? After many years of research on blueberry antioxidants and their potential benefits for the nervous system and for brain health, there is exciting new evidence that blueberries can improve memory. In a study involving older adults (with an average age of 76 years), 12 weeks of daily blueberry consumption was enough to improve scores on two different tests of cognitive function including memory.

While participants in the study consumed blueberries in the form of juice, three-quarters of a pound of blueberries were used to make each cup of juice. As participants consumed between 2 to 2-1/2 cups each day, the participants actually received a very plentiful amount of berries. The authors of this study were encouraged by the results and suggested that blueberries might turn out to be beneficial, not only for improvement of memory, but for slowing down or postponing the onset of other cognitive problems frequently associated with aging.[3]

Are you ready to boost your defense against Dementia and Alzheimer's with blueberries?

Strategy: Go to the market and stock up with fresh or frozen blueberries; plan for four to five servings a week. With new evidence that blueberries can improve memory, everyone will want to have their turn mixing up a special snack or dessert with those blueberries.

Suggestions:

- For a nutritious breakfast, add blueberries to non-fat Greek yogurt with chopped walnuts for a tasty crunch.
- Add fresh or dried blueberries to high fiber cereals.
- Add blueberries to baked cookies and muffins for lunch bag treats.

13 Super Brain Foods

Feeding your brain super brain foods is easy once you know what foods to add to your daily menus. Don't get overwhelmed about where to start.

The first step is to commit to a healthier lifestyle and focus on feeding your brain foods to help prevent the risk of dementia.

The second step is to shop for your favorite brain foods. I found it easier to start with just a few from the super brain foods list. My favorite breakfast menu is chopped walnuts with fresh blueberries or sliced strawberries stirred into non-fat Greek yogurt high in protein. Also, I drink hot or iced green tea.

The third, fourth, fifth and remaining steps will fall into place as you introduce more brain foods into your daily meal plan.

Here Is a List of 13 Super Brain Foods

Fish: Salmon, Anchovies, Mackerel, Tuna

Awash with nutrients, cold-water fish like salmon are a good source of Omega-3 Fatty Acids, which play an important role in strengthening synapses in your brain, strengthening brain function, and memory. One concern that many have about consuming fish are the levels of mercury that accumulate through the food chain and reside in salmon.

To avoid contaminates, experts recommend eating wild salmon. Wild Salmon is also an excellent source of EPA (eicosapentaenoic acid) and DHA (docosahexaenoic acid), two potent Omega-3 Fatty Acids that douse inflammation. Sardines, anchovies, and mackerel are also packed with brain-healthy omega-3s but have lower levels of mercury that may be found in other fish. They're easy to find canned in grocery stores and you can easily make them an ingredient in snacks and meals.

Turmeric

The Asian spice, Turmeric, is commonly found in pre-mixed curry powder and contains a powerful, non-toxic compound called curcumin. Studies found that turmeric's anti-inflammatory effects are on par with many potent drugs yet has none of their side effects, although we do not recommend substituting anything in place of a doctor's advice. In studies, Turmeric upregulates LDL receptor activity.

Mushrooms

For thousands of years, the Chinese have revered mushrooms, specifically Shiitake, Cordyceps, and Reishi, for their immune-boosting properties. Mushrooms may reduce platelet aggregation, increase blood flow, and supports lower cholesterol levels.

Avocado

Many consider avocadoes to be the food of the gods. This nutrient-packed fruit (yes, it's technically a fruit) is high in monostearate fat, which helps lower cholesterol and improve blood flow. Since the brain uses 20% of all oxygen the body consumes, it's vital to have healthy blood flow to carry oxygen and nutrients to the brain. Avocados are a good source for Omega-3 Fatty Acids and Vitamin E, which functions as an antioxidant and promotes healthy brain activity.

Nuts

Researchers have linked tree nuts to a decreased risk of many diseases. Now there is evidence that they also improve cognition. Most have high concentrations of Vitamin E, B Vitamins, antioxidants, magnesium, minerals and Omega-3s. All of them support the nervous system.

The walnut's shape resembles a brain, so why shouldn't it be a brain food? It is! Rich in both Omega-3 Fatty Acids and antioxidants, walnuts offer a variety of benefits for brain health. Since Omega-3 Fatty Acids are typically found in meats, walnuts provide a great non-meat alternative. They can help you concentrate and protect your brain against the effects of aging. Walnuts have also been shown to improve mood by influencing the brain's serotonin levels. For those who suffer from depression, insomnia, or related issues, walnuts may be a helpful food to munch on.

Almonds may help save your memory. In studies on laboratory mice, the rodents rendered temporarily amnesiac were more apt to remember their way around a maze 24 hours later if they first consumed an almond paste. The evidence suggests that almonds slow the decline in cognitive abilities linked to Alzheimer's disease. Investigators attribute the memory effects to the presence of the essential amino acid phenylalanine and L-carnitine. It is believed to boost neurotransmitters essential to memory.

Brazil nuts can spare the obese the vascular damage associated with adiposity. An excess of fat tissue stimulates low-grade inflammation and oxidative stress, both of which can lead to cardiovascular disease.

Brazil nuts improved microcirculation, lowered cholesterol levels, and normalized blood lipid profiles without causing weight gain in 17 obese female adolescents. The high levels of unsaturated fatty acids and bioactive substances (selenium, phenolic compounds, folate, magnesium among them) combat inflammation.

Green Tea

China's favorite drink has been shown to provide many benefits for memory and spatial learning and may impact cellular mechanisms in the brain. The organic chemical, EGCG (epigallocatechin-3 gallate) that is also found in green tea extract, is a key property of green tea and is a known antioxidant. EGCG is also found to boost the production of neural progenitor cells, which like stems cells can adapt, or differentiate, into various types of cells. In laboratory studies, EGCG enhances learning and memory by improving object and spatial memory.

Seeds: Flax, Chia, Hemp, Sesame

These small seeds provide big benefits for both the body and the brain. They are an even more potent source of Omega-3 Fatty Acids than walnuts. Also a good source of B Vitamins, eating flaxseeds can be a great way to give your brain cells what they need for improved cognitive function and memory.

Flaxseed is also a source of manganese, which acts as a powerful antioxidant. It's best to grind flaxseed before eating it since the body has difficulty absorbing the seed's nutrients when left in its natural state.

Chia seeds are a super-food that the ancient Mayans and Aztecs heavily relied upon. These seeds are packed with Omega-3 Fatty Acids and contain more antioxidants than blueberries. Add chia seeds to your diet for improved concentration, memory, mood, and protection against degenerative diseases like Alzheimer's. Sesame and hemp seeds contain plant sterols that help modulate the immune system.

Quinoa

Quinoa is an all-around good grain. It makes up a complete protein, containing all nine of the essential amino acids. Quinoa is also an excellent source of iron, which is needed to produce energy for the brain's neurons. It is also rich in riboflavin (or Vitamin B2), which is another important energy source.

Since the brain consumes such a large amount of the body's energy, it's important to eat the right foods to supply it.

Riboflavin also functions as an antioxidant, helping to protect cells from damage caused by free radicals.

Cruciferous Vegetables

Cruciferous vegetables like **broccoli, arugula, kale, spinach, collard greens, Brussels sprouts, cauliflower, bok choy, garden cress, and cabbage,** may not be considered the world's best tasting foods, especially by kids, but they have become highly regarded for being great sources of nutrients and dietary fiber. They are rich in Vitamin K, which has been shown to prevent arterial calcification in the brain, which may be linked to Alzheimer 's disease. Vitamin K also plays a role in creating important fats that the brain needs to perform properly.

Broccoli also contains sulforaphane that helps the body get rid of potentially carcinogenic compounds. In studies, broccoli, red cabbage and sulforaphane have been shown to reduce inflammation and oxidative stress.

Sweet Potato

A good complex carbohydrate, it's also a reliable source of beta-carotene, manganese, Vitamin B6 and C as well as dietary fiber. Combined, these are powerful antioxidants that support inflammation in the body.

Berries: There Is No Bad Berry

Adding berries to your diet can help your brain better process information to stay mentally sharp. Blackberries, blueberries, goji berries, strawberries, and cranberries are loaded up with polyphenols and antioxidants. These berries can help reduce inflammation in brain cells, making it easier for them to talk to each other. Polyphenols found in blackberries also help reduce accumulation of toxins in the brain.

Some evidence suggests blueberries, strawberries and cranberries can improve metabolic syndrome through lessoning inflammation.

Extra Virgin Olive Oil

Olive oil is a great source of monounsaturated fats, which have been shown to slow brain aging. Virgin olive oil is Mediterranean's secret to longevity. Its rich supply of polyphenols protects the heart and blood vessels from inflammation.

The monounsaturated fats in olive oil are also turned into anti-inflammatory agents by the body that can lower occurrences of asthma and rheumatoid arthritis.

Water

Don't forget this important nutrient. Water makes up 85% of brain weight. A study in Neurology found that dehydration decreases brain volume, and rehydration increases cerebral volume significantly.[4]

Other Brain Foods

When planning meals and snacks to prevent or lower the risk of dementia, there are many good brain foods from which to choose.

It is recommended that we eat more of the "protective foods" which are listed below. A daily intake of these healthy foods is also going to help improve our overall health status.

As we eat more of the brain foods, we will also need to begin to let go of unhealthy foods, some of which are listed below.

Brain Food: Diet Can Help Prevent Dementia after Age 50-Eating right in midlife may prevent dementia later on, according to a new doctoral thesis published by the University of Eastern Finland.

Results indicated those who consistently consumed healthy foods at the average age of 50 had a nearly 90% lower risk of dementia in a 14-year follow-up study compared to those who did not eat healthfully.

Researchers used a healthy diet index based on eating a variety of foods. "Healthy" foods included vegetables, berries/fruits, fish and unsaturated fats from milk products and spreads.

"Unhealthy" foods included sausages, eggs, salty fish, sugary drinks, desserts/candy and saturated fats from milk products and spreads.

Participants were between 39 and 64 years old, and 65 to 79 years old at the study baseline and follow-up, respectively.

While 2,000 participants were involved in the initial study, 1,449 completed the follow-up.

Eating a large amount of saturated fats was linked to decreased cognitive function and increased dementia risk. Those who eat a diet high in saturated fats and carry the epsilon 4 variant of the apolipoprotein E (ApoE) gene are also at risk.

This gene is a risk factor for Alzheimer's disease. "Even those who are genetically susceptible can at least delay the onset of the disease by favoring vegetable oils, oil-based spreads and fatty fish in their diet," says doctoral thesis author Margo Eskelinen, MSc.

The thesis was based on the population-based Finnish Cardiovascular Risk Factors, Aging and Incidence of Dementia (CAIDE) study.

The Alzheimer's Association recommends increasing intake of "protective foods" to maintain a healthy brain.

These include dark-skinned fruits and vegetables such as prunes, raisins, red grapes, plums, blueberries, cherries, broccoli, spinach, kale, onion, red bell pepper, beets and eggplant.

Nuts such as almonds, walnuts and pecans are also recommended, as are cold-water fish such as trout, salmon, tuna, mackerel and halibut.

Increasing intake of Vitamins such as C, E, folate and B12 is also considered helpful.

Study results were published in the International Journal of Geriatric Psychiatry, Dementia and Geriatric Cognitive Disorders and Journal of Alzheimer's Disease.[5]

Shopping List with Super Brain Foods.

Download and print copy of the shopping list on the following page to use as a guide when you shop.

Download from: SandraPye.com/register

Continue to take one step at a time to feed your brain the foods needed to prevent the risk of dementia.

<u>**Shopping List with Super Brain Foods**</u>

Super Brain Foods *

BERRIES / FRUIT

☐ Avocado * ☐ Blackberries * ☐ Blueberries *

☐ Cranberries * ☐ Goji Berries * ☐ Red Seedless Grapes *

☐ Strawberries * ☐ Fresh Fruit ☐ Lemons (or 100% bottled lemon Juice)

BEVERAGES ☐ Green Tea * ☐ Orange Juice ☐ Water*

BREAD ☐ (100% Whole Grain loaf) ___________ other

CONDIMENTS / SIDES / OTHER

☐ Brown Rice ☐ Hollandaise Sauce (drizzle on asparagus & broccoli)

☐ Quinoa * ☐ Salad dressing ☐ Turmeric *

DAIRY ☐ Non-fat Greek yogurt (prefer: **OIKO** 5.3 oz. in black ctn.) also Official Yogurt of NFL!

FISH ☐ Anchovies * ☐ Mackerel * ☐ Salmon * ☐ Trout * ☐ Tuna * ________ other

MEATS / POULTRY

☐ Chicken ☐ Chicken tenders ☐ canned chicken (for chicken salad)

☐ Turkey ☐ Turkey burger patties ☐ baked turkey breast –deli

☐ (Rack of Ribs to grill or from deli already cooked) _________ Other

NUTS ☐ Walnuts * ☐ Pecans * ☐ Brazil Nuts * _________ Other

OILS ☐ Extra Virgin Olive Oil *

☐ Coconut Oil* (non-hydrogenated)

SEEDS ☐ Flax * ☐ Sesame * ☐ Hemp * ☐ Chia *

VEGETABLES

☐ Asparagus * ☐ Beets * ☐ Broccoli * ☐ Brussels Sprout *

☐ Butterbeans ☐ Cabbage * ☐ Carrots ☐ Cauliflower *

☐ Collard Greens * ☐ Corn on the Cob ☐ Cream Corn ☐ Cucumbers

☐ Carrots ☐ Green Salads * ☐ Kale * ☐ Mushrooms *

☐ Peas ☐ Pole Beans ☐ Spinach * ☐ Sweet Potato *

☐ Stewed Tomatoes (Canned) ☐ Tomatoes ______ other

References:

1. Sacks, F. Dr. (2007, June 19). The Expert: Omega-3 Fatty Acids. Retrieved from www.hsph.harvard.edu/nutritionsource/2007/06/19/ask-the-expert-omega-3-fatty-Acids

2. Staff of FCA Medical Publishing. (2012). Alzheimer's & Memory loss. In *Super Abundant Health* (pp. 7-26). Peachtree city, GA: FC&A publishing.

3. The George Mateljan Foundation. World's Healthiest Foods. Available at: http://www.whfoods.org/ What's New and Beneficial About Blueberries? Retrieved January 30, 2017

4. Nature's Sunshine Products, Inc. (n.d.). 13 super brain foods. Retrieved from http://www.naturessunshine.com/

5. Huffington Post. (2012, March 3). Brain food: Diet can help prevent dementia after age 50. Retrieved from http://www.huffingtonpost.ca/2014/03/12/brain-food n 4948811.html

Photo Credits:

- Salmon image - rusak-canstockphoto.com
- Brain image - maxxyustas-canstockphoto.com
- Walnut image - matteobragaglio-canstockphoto.com
- Blueberries image - kalozzolak-canstockphoto.com

CHAPTER 4

PHYSICAL ACTIVITIES

Can I Stop My Brain from Shrinking?

YES, you CAN stop your brain from shrinking.

You may not know this, but there is a PROTEIN that triggers brain cell growth.

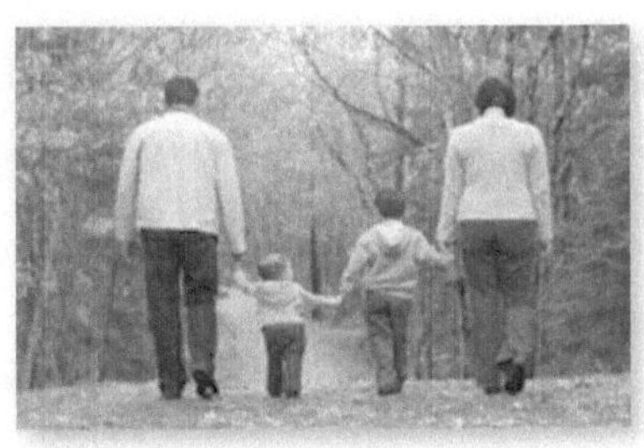

I know you are already thinking "Where can I get this stuff? I want it now!"

The bad news first – it's not available for sale anywhere.

Now the good news, it's FREE!

That's right. All you have to do to get it is to walk at least 3 times a week, 30 minutes each time.

The physical activity causes increased production of this special PROTEIN in the body.

- *For added benefit, walk 2 more days per week for 30 minutes to meet the Surgeon General's requirements of walking 150 minutes per week for diabetes prevention.*

That's it.

I gave you the 'secret' right up front.

But, continue reading to get the whole story.

http://SandraPye.com/contact

Cardio Exercises Build New Brain Cells
Walking Briskly and Pedaling a Bicycle

Walking Briskly

Participating in physical fitness activities causes you to increase production of brain-derived neurotropic factor--a protein that triggers brain cell growth. Also, by participating in physical activity – like walking 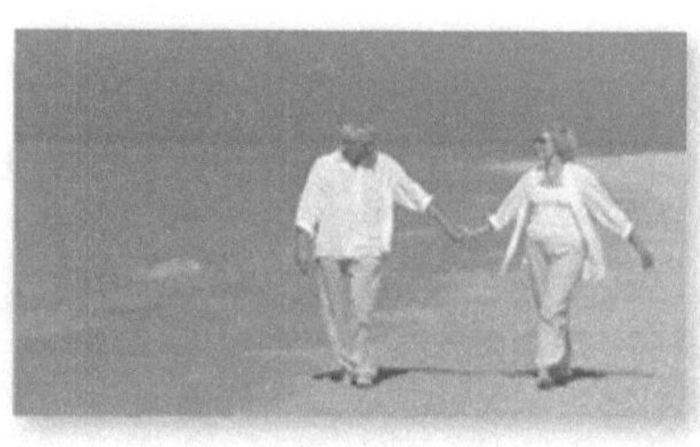 – it causes you to maintain good circulation to ensure a steady supply of nutrients and oxygen to the brain.

A recent study showed evidence when sedentary retirees started walking three times a week, their brains were measured by MRI scans six months later and had grown by an average of 3%. That is roughly the equivalent of taking three years off the age of their brains. [1]

Pedaling a Bicycle and a Stationary Bike

Exercises that grow your mind are like fertilizer for your brain. All those hours spent turning your cranks creates rich capillary beds not only in your quads and glutes, but also in your gray matter. More blood vessels in your 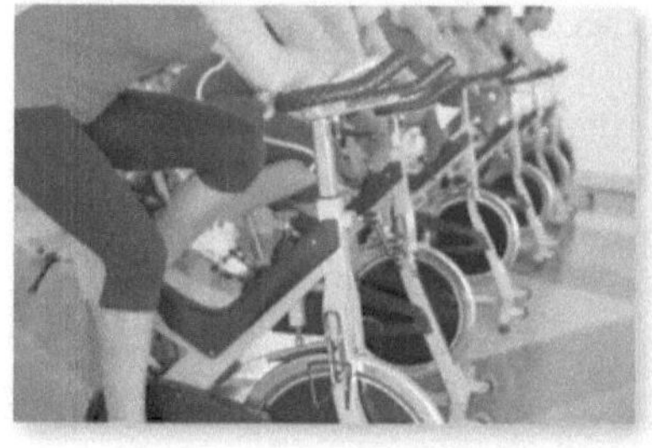 brain and muscles mean more oxygen and nutrients to help them work. When you pedal, you also force more nerve cells to fire. As these neurons light up, they intensify the creation of proteins like brain-derived neurotrophic factor (BDNF) and a compound called noggin (yes, really), which promote the formation of new brain cells. The result: You double or triple the production of neurons—literally building your brain. You also release neurotransmitters (the messengers between your brain cells) so all those cells, new and old, can communicate with each other for better, faster functioning. That's a pretty profound benefit to cyclists. [2]

Run on a Treadmill for More-Demanding Exercise

In a study published in Perceptual and Motor Skills, women performed 20% better on memory tests after running on a treadmill than they did before exercising. They also increased problem-solving abilities by 20%. The intensity of your workout makes a difference, too. A study in Neurobiology of Learning and Memory found that people learned vocabulary words 20% faster after 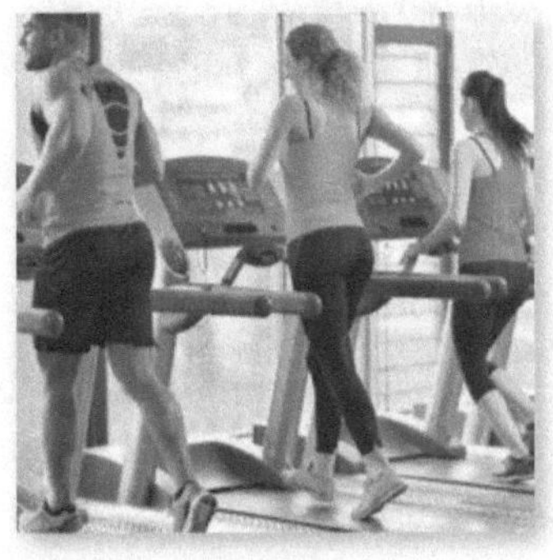 intense exercise than after low-intensity activity. Those who did more-demanding exercise had a bigger spike in their brains' levels of BDNF, dopamine, and epinephrine afterward. So, the more you challenge your body, the more your gray matter benefits.[3]

Walking or Outdoor Cycling May Not Be Possible Some Days

There will be days you can't get outside due to bad weather, unexpected family emergencies, sickness, etc. On these days, cycle on a stationary bike in the comfort of home or walk inside a local mall to stay on schedule.

I didn't want to skip days on my walking schedule and wanted a backup plan ready. I took my antique Sears stationary bike out of storage and spruced it up with a glossy white paint job and added a comfortable seat. I would like a brand new stationary bike with all the bells and whistles, but I have become attached to this oldie for now. The cycle is in plain view of my comfy chair as a gentle reminder to add more exercise to my schedule.

Stationary cycling time is used to catch up with the news on TV. And the madder I get with the grim news reports, the faster I pedal to break a sweat and gain more health benefits!

However, you need to push yourself to get outside and exercise as often as possible for fresh air and sunshine and to mix and mingle with others to keep your communication skills active.

If only I had known then, what I know now...

I would have insisted Mother get on a regular 30-minute walking schedule at least three days a week.

Even if we had to sign up the grandkids to walk with her, it would have been worth it to trigger brain cell growth.

With a stationary bike in her home she could have kept active on days she didn't walk, and thus, prevented her memory loss and confusion.

Strategy: Now that you know a 'special secret' about what walking can do for your brain, you will more likely be interested in walking for your regular exercise. When I walk now, I think about all the 'bells and whistles and wires coming alive' inside my brain in preparation to make new cells, and that makes me happy!

For a person to be able to increase production of a protein that triggers brain cell growth just by walking 30 minutes a day at least 3 times a week is awesome. This is a crucial step to help prevent or reduce the risk of dementia.

Suggestions: Follow these ten simple steps if you are ready to start walking or cycling.

1. First, discuss your current health and exercise plans with your doctor to ensure that it meets with their approval.

2. Commit to DO THIS at least 3 times per week for 30 minutes each time, increase to five times per week for diabetes prevention.

3. Pick a day to start.

4. ***Choose a safe location to walk or bicycle.***

5. Wear comfortable walking shoes.

6. Carry a small bottle of water.

7. Take your cell phone *in case of an emergency.*

8. Grab your hat and sunglasses.

9. If you need extra motivation, convince a family member, friend or neighbor to join you.

10. GET STARTED!

Get Involved - Walk to End Alzheimer's.

Held annually in more than 600 communities nationwide, Walk to End Alzheimer's is the world's largest event to raise awareness and funds for Alzheimer's care, support and research. https://act.alz.org

How to Participate in Three Easy Steps

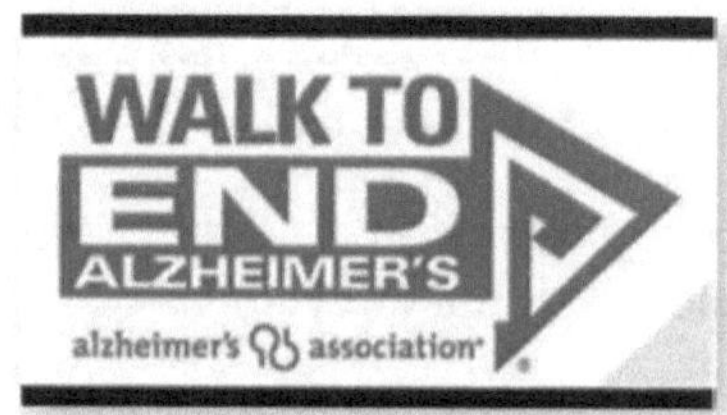

1. **Find a walk** in your community.

2. **Register** as a team captain, team member, or individual.

3. **Start fundraising** and raising awareness.

For more information, Walk to End Alzheimer's.

References:

1. Bottom Line Publications. (2012). Your brain unlimited. Retrieved from http://www.bottomline.com

2. Asp, K. (n.d.). How exercise boosts your brain power. Retrieved from http://www.active.com/fitness/articles/how-exercise-boosts-your-brainpower

Photo Credits:

-   Family of four walking – talltrevor – canstockphoto.com
-   Couple walking on beach - Daren Baker-canstockphoto.com
-   Riders on Stationary Bikes – 20890758canstockphoto.com
-   Runners on Treadmills – 26009059canstockphoto.com

CHAPTER 5

MENTAL ACTIVITIES

Take the Challenge - Generate New Brain Cells and Have Fun Doing It!

Scientific research shows that stimulating brain activity will generate new brain cells when done regularly. Commit to keeping your brain active by engaging in a favored mental activity 1-2 hours daily. Some may 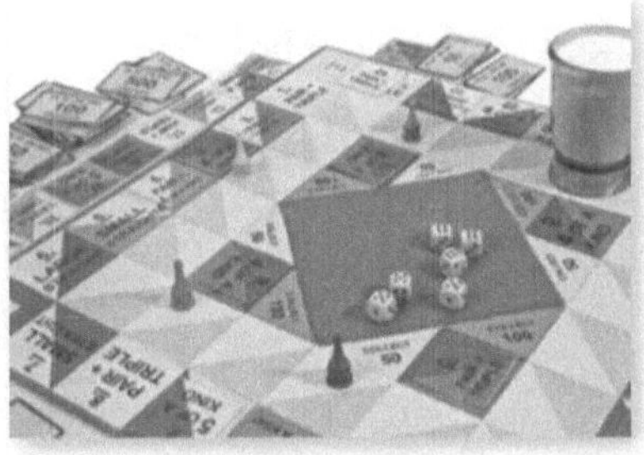 say you are just wasting your time playing brain games; ignore them and continue with your fun. We must nurture our brain every day with lots of fun and TLC (tender loving care) to avoid a possible downward spiral of dementia.

Fading memory and declining cognitive skills are often blamed on advancing age. But, unhealthful habits such as sedentary lifestyle, chronic illnesses, depression, alcohol, and poor choices of food cause more harm to the brain 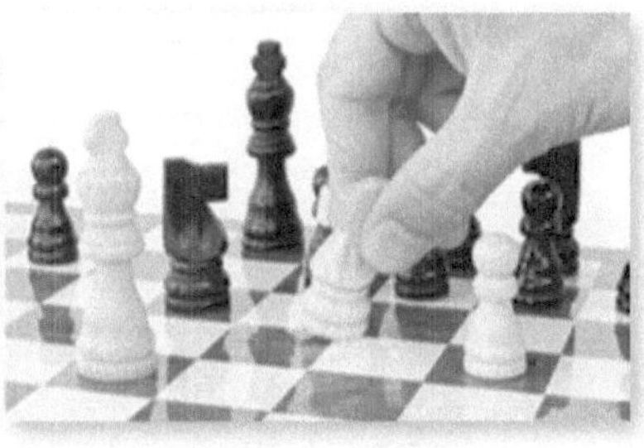 than advancing age. A growing body of scientific research suggests including a steady dose of mental activities/challenges in your daily schedule such as brain activity games. Scientists used to say we had a finite number of brain cells, but now research has indicated that we are able to generate new brain cells (neurons) and connections (synapses) between them. One of the best ways to stimulate brain activity is to learn new skills.[1]

Here Are a Few Suggestions to Help You Get Started:

1. Visit your local library. Check out an instructional CD or book that teaches a foreign language or special skill you want to learn.

2. Chess, bridge, backgammon, and other board games provide a good brain workout.

3. Crossword puzzles, word search puzzles, and the number-placement activity Sudoku give your brain a good 'think and solve' workout.

4. Check out other books of interest in bookstores. If you can't think of a good book to read, scan the bookshelves in the *special interest* section to find a book title that sparks an interest.

5. Schedule time with family and friends for fun and happy interaction time. A few doses of laughter are good medicine to help maintain a healthy brain.

6. If you work, get outside at lunch for a brisk walk and/or eat lunch in the park. This is important if you work a sedentary job. If you commute to work via public transportation, use that time to play brain games on your Smartphone, tablet, or, other electronic device.

Interact with Friends and Family to Reduce Your Risk of Dementia

I have many special memories of quality time spent vacationing with my family and parents.

My parents loved to travel to the mountains. Many summers we traveled together to spend time in the Great Smoky Mountains. As mealtimes came around, we searched for picnic tables and campsites near a creek or mountain stream so the kids could wade in the creek and walk on the large, smooth rocks in the water. Dad grilled burgers, and Mother always made homemade potato salad and sliced homegrown tomatoes to round out the meal.

Several times we encountered black bears. Once we had to jump in the car and give the bear our feast! Though exciting to be that close to a huge bear, we were happy it was from the safety of our car.

One year we ventured in the opposite direction to Key West, Florida. The most memorable event of the trip involved crossing the old and narrow seven-mile long bridge across the ocean to Key West Island. Terrified of bridges, I laid on the back seat when we crossed it.

I learned about the bridge when we arrived in Miami while visiting with my sister-in-law.

Mother wanted to go to Key West, but never mentioned the bridge. I told everyone we were not going any further south on this vacation. Mother said, "Oh, yes we are going to Key West in the morning. I traveled this far (10 hours) to see Key West, and we are going tomorrow." Mother had spoken. End of discussion.

Those years spent vacationing with our children and my parents are among my most precious memories today.

Mother's Mental Stamina While Dad Was Alive

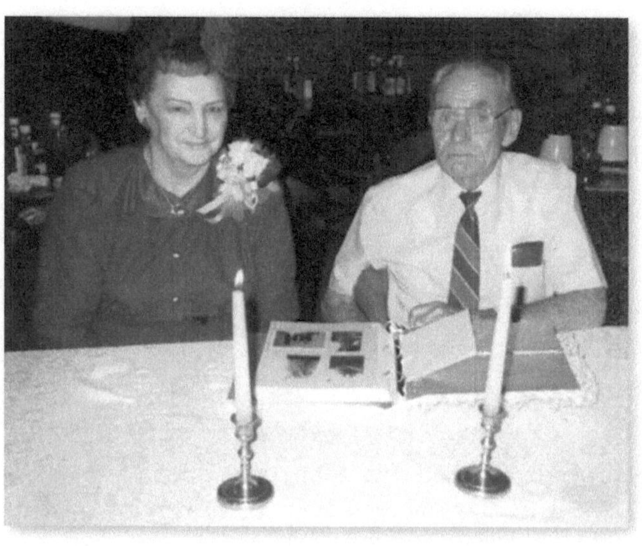

Mother and Dad at their 50th Anniversary Party at the Golden Corral.

Mother and Dad enjoyed a long and happy marriage and were together 53 years. They worked together as a team on our farm to provide for our family.

Mother was Dad's primary caregiver during and after his heart and lung surgeries which were only eight weeks apart.

His heart surgery was first with four bypasses at 70 years of age. Then he had lung surgery to remove part of a lung due to cancer.

Radiation treatments focused on the cancer site daily for the next 30 days.

The cancer continued to grow; too weak for another surgery, Dad passed away six months later.

After that, Mother became overwhelmed with loneliness and exhaustion. She told me that she thought life was over with Dad gone and no longer felt joy in her life. Soon after, we saw bits and pieces of memory loss and confusion in Mother's interactions with us.

She stopped going to church because she missed him sitting by her side, and the old familiar church hymns only made her more emotional. When she stopped going to church, she lost social interaction with her close lady friends in the church.

Mother had shared a close relationship with her two sisters and two sisters-in-law. Sadly, one sister and one sister-in-law passed away before Dad did.

In her emotional state of mind, grieving and depressed, she missed the special camaraderie once shared with friends and family.

We tried to help Mother grieve while we also grieved the loss of our wonderful and loving Dad. He was our rock! This is one example of how life events can affect memory loss and cause a decline in cognitive skills. It can turn a person's world upside down.

Social Interaction - People Are Good Medicine

Social interaction can be measured by how often people talk on the phone with friends and family, how often they attend social outings, and how many people they can trust with their most private feelings and concerns. Socializing has a protective effect on the brain because it's a form of mental exercise. Not only does interacting with people stimulate the brain, but it can also keep you sharp, because dealing with people can be challenging.

Strong social ties have been associated with lower blood pressure and longer life expectancies. And having no social ties is believed to be an independent risk factor for cognitive decline in older persons. U.S. researchers found that talking to another person for 10 minutes a day improves memory and test scores. They found that socializing was just as effective as more traditional kinds of mental exercise in boosting memory and intellectual performance. They also found that the higher the level of social interaction, the better the cognitive functioning.

Social interaction included getting together or having phone chats with relatives, friends and neighbors. In a study of more than 2,800 people ages 65 or older, Harvard researchers found that those with at least five social ties -- such as church groups, social groups, regular visits, or phone calls with family and friends - were less likely to suffer cognitive decline than those with no social ties. [2]

Strategy: You learned that we can generate new brain cells by engaging in mental activities one to two hours daily. Think about the mental activities you enjoy the most and try to set a special time for them on your daily calendar. Make it a priority to interact with friends and family daily to keep you sharp and maintain your social skills.

Suggestions:

Do you have a passion for something you always wanted to do or something you never had time to explore? It could be a long-time desire to return to college and finally, get that degree.

"It is never too late to be what you might have been."

– George Eliot.

- Start a genealogy study and track your great, great, grandparents and learn more about your family history.
- Mark a daily one to two-hour time slot on your calendar: FT (Fun Time), to generate new brain cells.
- Collect your favorite brain workout games puzzles, board games, and interesting books at flea markets, yard sales, and even at your local Goodwill store. These 'outings' can be a fun activity to find these and other 'treasures.'

Suggestions for People in the Workforce:

- If you work or spend your lunch break eating at your desk, STOP!
- If your employer offers a company gym or gym membership, use it.
- Start a noon-hour workout session with your co-workers.
- Need alone time and fresh air? Search for parks or other recreational areas to spend work breaks.
- In bad weather, search for art galleries, bookstores or other interesting spots to stimulate your brain.
- Do something opposite your work duties to exercise your body and brain. A leisurely stroll is healthier than spending lunch breaks at your desk.

References:

1. Bottom Line Publications. (2012). Your Brain Unlimited. Retrieved from http://bottomlineinc.com/category/bottomlinehealth/

2. EMed Expert. (2009). How to boost brain power and memory. Retrieved July 2016, from http://www.emedexpert.com/tips/brain.shtml

Photo Credits:

- Monopoly game - Lynne Albright-canstockphoto.com
- Chess game - Faraways-canstockphoto.com

CHAPTER 6

WELLNESS

Get a Good Night's Sleep

Sleep Well to Prevent Dementia

Oh, what a sweet relief just to lay your head down on your cozy pillow at bedtime, snuggle under your favorite blanket, and settle into that perfect position for a wonderful night of sleep and rest. Two hours later, you are still tossing and turning, 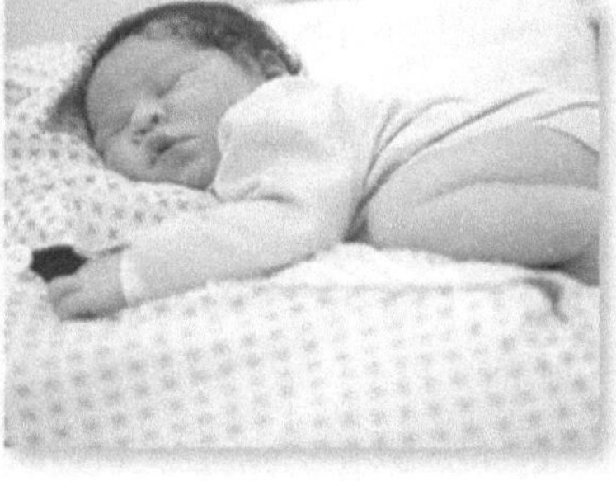 pillows are on the floor, covers twisted around you in a mess, and you are worn out. When will sleep come? Is this the scenario that you experience most nights?

For some, getting a good night's sleep isn't easy. Some people may suffer from interrupted sleep throughout the night, as with those who have sleep apnea. Individuals may suffer from insomnia, which becomes more common with age, while others may "sleep like a baby" most nights.

Try the steps below to improve your sleep habits. Be sure to get a good night's sleep each night to prevent or reduce your risk of dementia.

http://SandraPye.com/contact

5 Ways to Sleep More Soundly

Sleep plays a crucial role in your health, energy levels and everyday functioning. Observe your sleep patterns for a few weeks. Then try these five strategies for better sleep.

If you have trouble falling asleep or staying asleep, you're not alone. Many people struggle with sleep — and that's a problem since sleep plays a crucial role in your health, energy levels and ability to function at your best. Most adults require seven to eight hours of sleep each night to feel well-rested and energized each day.

If restless nights have become the norm for you, the first step toward getting better sleep is to observe your sleep patterns. Take note of how much you sleep each night, what factors contribute to your sleep or lack of it, how rested you feel the next morning, and how much energy you have throughout the day.

After observing your sleep patterns for one to two weeks, try the strategies below to help improve your sleep. Keep making adjustments until restless nights become a thing of the past.

1. ***Minimize light and sound.*** These two environmental factors can impact both your quality and quantity of sleep. Darkness causes your brain to release melatonin for a calming, sleepy effect. As a result, it's important to minimize your exposure to light before bedtime. Even the light from your computer, television or other devices might make it more difficult for you to fall asleep. Ban these devices from your bedroom and create a dark space by using blackout shades or an eye mask. Noise can also interfere with your ability to sleep. Try using a fan or a noise machine to block out unwanted noises.

2. ***Get comfortable.*** Adults spend about a third of their lives asleep, so it's worthwhile to invest in bedding that comforts and relaxes you. Before climbing into bed, try lowering your thermostat a few degrees. Your core temperature drops during rest, and keeping your room on the chilly side will aid in this natural temperature drop.

3. ***Keep a routine.*** Just like kids, adults sleep better when they have a bedtime routine. Doing the same thing before bed each night can help prepare your body for rest and condition your brain for sleep. Stick to activities that promote relaxation such as gentle stretching, journaling, reading or meditation.

4. ***Manage stress.*** How you handle stress can play a significant role in your ability to fall and stay asleep. While stress isn't all bad, when it turns into worry or anxiety, it can disrupt your sleep. If your busy mind keeps you up at night, try practicing stress management techniques before you go to bed. Experiment with aromatherapy, deep breathing, keeping a gratitude journal or meditation.

5. ***Get out of bed.*** If you find yourself lying in bed stressing about your inability to sleep, get out of bed and do something that will promote relaxation. This might be reading an uninteresting book, practicing a relaxation technique or focusing on your breathing. When you begin to feel drowsy, head back to bed.

Make sleep a priority. Even if you're already sleeping soundly, these tips can help. If you're not getting enough sleep, keep using these suggestions until you get the sleep you need to feel your best each day.[1]

Are you ready to make your perfect, or almost perfect, night-time sleep scenario come true?

Strategy: You read the suggestions above, commit to reevaluate your sleep patterns and sleep schedule. Observe your present sleep habits for a few nights and see what happens. The suggestions below should help you start a simple night-time journal.

Suggestions:

- Take a legal notepad and draw a line down the middle of the page. Title the first column with the heading: "*What Works*" and in the second column, "What *Doesn't Work.*" Keep the notepad and pen on the nightstand beside your bed. This is the start of your journal to help you find solutions that will help you get the quality of sleep your brain needs every night.
- Record *what works* and *doesn't work* to end bad habits and add healthy behaviors to create a more comfortable, cozy "sleep nest." You may need to add a better pillow or a warmer, cozier blanket. Check room temperature and the noise level. Do you need soft music playing OR NOT? Did you sleep too much during the day? Did you eat or drink too much or too late before bed? Make yourself aware of these items as you make notes in your journal.

Try to journal for at least a week or more. It will help you to focus on your environment and may help you improve your sleep routine.

Stop Smoking

People who smoke don't like being told smoking is harmful to their health and that they should quit; they already know.

It's clear that smokers enjoy the smoking process as much as some folks LOVE their morning coffee. Some smokers describe a sense of relaxation while others experience a sense of euphoria.

To understand why people smoke, I compared a person's cigarette addiction to my 'must have' early morning cup of coffee. When I wake up, I don't want to talk or do anything until I sit in my comfortable chair and take my time sipping and savoring the hot and creamy deliciousness-until the last drop. I would get agitated if people told me I should stop drinking my morning cup of coffee because caffeine is not good for me

With that said, I have a better understanding why it's not so easy to just quit. It seems a person must be at a crossroad in their life and ready to make an important lifestyle choice to smoke that LAST cigarette, or NOT.

As a final note, this information on the negative effects of smoking and inhaling nicotine may help smokers quit and non-smokers to remain non-smokers.

How Nicotine Affects Body Chemistry

When inhaled, *nicotine travels to the brain quickly* (within 10 seconds) and attaches to receptors where the neurotransmitter acetylcholine would normally dock. This starts a chain of chemical reactions that influence numerous bodily functions.

Most smokers are familiar with the feeling of a racing heart and/ or shallow breathing when they smoke. Adrenaline, the 'fight or flight' hormone, is responsible for this. When nicotine reaches the brain, adrenaline is released, increasing heart rate, blood pressure, and restricting blood flow to the heart.

Adrenaline also tells the body to move excess glucose into the bloodstream. At the same time, nicotine hinders the release of insulin from the pancreas, which would remove excess sugar from the blood. The result is that smokers are often in a state of hyperglycemia, meaning they have more sugar in their blood than is normal.

High blood sugar dampens hunger, and this is a contributing factor for the appetite-suppressant effects of nicotine.

How Nicotine Hurts Your Health

Research has uncovered a link between nicotine and vascular smooth muscle cell damage, contributing to the formation of plaques that lead to heart disease.

Nicotine slows the production of bone-producing cells called osteoblasts. This prolongs healing when bones are broken.

Nicotine inhibits apoptosis, a process that removes unwanted cells in the body (programmed cell death). Since some of the cells targeted by apoptosis are mutations that may become cancerous in the future, inhibiting this important function may contribute to life-threatening diseases.

Smoking is a known risk factor for degenerative disc disease. Nicotine and carbon monoxide in cigarette smoke hinder spinal disc cells from absorbing vital nutrients in blood, which in turn leads to premature dehydration and degeneration of spinal discs. Nicotine is among the most toxic of all poisons and is highly addictive.

It is a mistake to think that using nicotine in a form that doesn't involve cigarettes is harmless. Products like smokeless tobacco and electronic cigarettes may be considered less harmful when compared to cigarette smoking, but they carry considerable health hazards as well. And don't forget, while nicotine addiction is actively engaged, ex-smokers are at a heightened risk for a full-fledged smoking relapse. Don't settle for less than you deserve. Recovery from nicotine addiction takes some work, but it is doable and so rewarding. [2]

Strategy: We have not covered all the reasons that smoking is harmful to our health and how it increases the risk of dementia. There are more than enough reasons listed to help you make a healthy choice about smoking. If you do not currently smoke, don't start.

Suggestions:

- When you are ready to quit smoking, visit this website: tobaccofree.org/quitting.htm. This excellent FREE guide will help you to quit. They have the resources needed to help you on your journey from the beginning to completion of your goal and beyond.

Keep Blood Pressure at a Healthy Level

High blood pressure can lead to stroke and heart disease and can increase risk of dementia. Living a healthy lifestyle can keep blood pressure in check. Visit your family physician as soon as possible if you are having immediate issues and concerns.

When high blood pressure is under control, other health problems improve also. There are many ways HBP can be controlled without medication.

See tips below:

10 Ways to Control High Blood Pressure Without Medication

By making these 10 lifestyle changes, you can lower your blood pressure and reduce your risk of heart disease without medication:

1. Lose extra pounds and watch your waistline

2. Exercise regularly

3. Eat a healthy diet

4. Reduce sodium in your diet

5. Limit the amount of alcohol you drink

6. Quit smoking

7. Cut back on caffeine

8. Reduce your stress

9. Monitor your blood pressure at home and see your doctor regularly

10. Get support

Lifestyle plays an important role in treating your high blood pressure. If you successfully control your blood pressure with a healthy lifestyle, you might avoid, delay or reduce the need for medication. [3]

Complications of High Blood Pressure

Here's a look at the complications high blood pressure can cause when it's not effectively controlled.

Damage to Your Arteries

Healthy arteries are flexible, strong and elastic. Their inner lining is smooth so that blood flows freely, supplying vital organs and tissues with adequate nutrients and oxygen. If you have high blood pressure, the increased pressure of blood flowing through your arteries gradually can cause a variety of problems, including the following:

Narrowing Arteries

High blood pressure can damage the cells of your arteries' inner lining. That launches a cascade of events that make artery walls thick and stiff, a disease called arteriosclerosis (ahr-teer-e-o-skluh-ROE-sis), or hardening of the arteries. Fats from your diet enter your bloodstream, pass through the damaged cells and collect to start atherosclerosis (ath-ur-o-skluh-ROE-sis). These changes can affect arteries throughout your body, blocking blood flow to your heart, kidneys, brain, arms and legs. The damage can cause many problems, including chest pain (angina), heart attack, heart failure, kidney failure, stroke, blocked arteries in your legs or arms (peripheral artery disease), eye damage, and aneurysms.

Aneurysm

Over time, the constant pressure of blood moving through a weakened artery can cause a section of its wall to enlarge and form a bulge (aneurysm). An aneurysm (AN-yoo-riz-um) can potentially rupture and cause life-threatening internal bleeding. Aneurysms can form in any artery throughout your body, but they're most common in the aorta, your body's largest artery.

Damage to Your Heart

Your heart pumps blood to your entire body. Uncontrolled high blood pressure can damage your heart in a number of ways, such as:

- ***Coronary Artery Disease***
  Coronary artery disease affects the arteries that supply blood to your heart muscle. Arteries narrowed by coronary artery disease don't allow blood to flow freely through your arteries. When blood can't flow freely to your heart, you can experience chest pain, a heart attack or irregular heart rhythms (arrhythmias).

- ***Enlarged Left Heart***
  High blood pressure forces your heart to work harder than necessary in order to pump blood to the rest of your body. This causes the left ventricle to thicken or stiffen (left ventricular hypertrophy). These changes limit the ventricle's ability to pump blood to your body. This condition increases your risk of heart attack, heart failure and sudden cardiac death.

Heart Failure

Over time, the strain on your heart caused by high blood pressure can cause your heart muscle to weaken and work less efficiently. Eventually, your overwhelmed heart simply begins to wear out and fail. Damage from heart attacks adds to this problem.

Damage to Your Brain

Just like your heart, your brain depends on a nourishing blood supply to work properly and survive. High blood pressure can cause several problems, including the following:

Transient Ischemic Attack (TIA)

Sometimes called a mini stroke, a transient ischemic (is-KEE-mik) attack is a brief, temporary disruption of blood supply to your brain. It's often caused by atherosclerosis or a blood clot — both of which can arise from high blood pressure. A transient ischemic attack is often a warning that you're at risk of a full-blown stroke.

Stroke

A stroke occurs when part of your brain is deprived of oxygen and nutrients, causing brain cells to die. Uncontrolled high blood pressure can lead to stroke by damaging and weakening your brain's blood vessels, causing them to narrow, rupture or leak. High blood pressure can also cause blood clots to form in the arteries leading to your brain, blocking blood flow and potentially causing a stroke.

Dementia

Dementia is a brain disease resulting in problems with thinking, speaking, reasoning, memory, vision and movement. There are several causes of dementia. One cause, vascular dementia, can result from narrowing and blockage of the arteries that supply blood to the brain. It can also result from strokes caused by an interruption of blood flow to the brain. In either case, high blood pressure may be the culprit.

Mild Cognitive Impairment

Mild cognitive impairment is a transition stage between the changes in understanding and memory that come with aging and the more-serious problems caused by Alzheimer's disease. Like dementia, it can result from blocked blood flow to the brain when high blood pressure damages arteries. [4]

Strategy:

Take steps to control your blood pressure and avoid many complications. Also, visit your doctor if you are having problems.

Suggestions: Re-read *"10 ways to control blood pressure without medication"* and, note the steps you will need to put into action. Take action one step at a time to get your blood pressure under control.

References:

1. Peterson, S. M. (2017, December 7). 5 ways to sleep more soundly. Retrieved May 20, 2017, from.
    http://www.mayoclinic.org/healthy-lifestyle/adult-health/in-depth/five-ways-sleep-soundly/art-20267152

2. Crews, T. (n.d.). Important facts about nicotine you should know. Retrieved August 2016, from https://www.verywell.com/nicotine-facts-you-should-know-2825019

3. Mayo Clinic Staff. (2016, November 23). High blood pressure dangers: Hypertension's effects on your body - Mayo Clinic. Retrieved from http://www.mayoclinic.org/diseases-conditions/high-blood-pressure/in-depth/high-blood-pressure/art-20045868

4. Mayo Clinic Staff. (2016, September 9). High blood pressure (hypertension) - Mayo Clinic. Retrieved from http://www.mayoclinic.org/diseases-conditions/high-blood-pressure/basics/definition/con-20019580

Photo Credits:

- Sleeping baby - linmar-canstockphoto.com

SECTION IV

Promising Research

CHAPTER 7

COCONUT OIL AND MCT OIL MEDIUM CHAIN TRIGLYCERIDES

How Coconut Oil with MCT Oil Feeds and Nurtures Your Brain

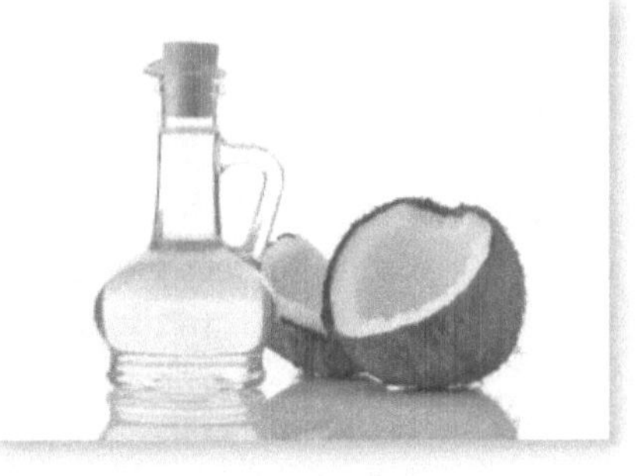

Coconut oil continues to be a hot topic about how it can help people with memory problems to think more clearly and restore memory loss. Who doesn't want this? Coconut oil is helping Alzheimer's patients get their life back and may help prevent Alzheimer's disease and other types of dementia.

I researched it to share what I found for those who are searching for hope to prevent or reduce the risk of dementia and for Alzheimer's patients to get their life back.

As I began my research on coconut oil, I was drawn to Dr. Mary Newport's findings on her website, CoconutKetones.com (Videos 1-6). At the time these videos were done, Mary Newport, MD had been a Neonatologist for 29 years and was also wife/caregiver to her husband, Steve. Steve began having symptoms at age 51 and was diagnosed with Alzheimer's disease at age 53. On her website, she tells her husband's story and their journey as she goes through these videos.[1]

In Dr. Newport's video interviews, she discusses searching for a product to help her husband Steve, who was diagnosed with early onset Alzheimer's disease at age 53 in 2003. She hoped to find a miraculous cure to help him 'hold on' to the memory capabilities he still had before it was too late for him to 'come back'.

Steve's condition continued to worsen into 2008; his personality slowly evaporated, and he smiled less. Since his diagnosis in 2003, he had taken two drugs made for Alzheimer's patients. However, these drugs only slow the progress and do nothing to reverse or improve the condition.

Dr. Newport learned that Alzheimer's is called diabetes of the brain or brain starvation. Certain areas of the brain are associated with getting glucose into the cells (glucose or sugar we all use for all the cells in our body). In Alzheimer's patients, glucose can't get into certain brain cells, and they die.

In May 2008, Dr. Newport saw an ad for two new drugs scheduled for testing in clinical trials. She had to choose which screening he should sign up for if he qualified for both trials. After researching the risks and benefits of the drugs, she found a patent application on a third medical food which noted improvement seen in their studies of MCT Oil. Medium Chain Triglycerides Oil (MCT Oil), an active ingredient in Coconut Oil, is partly converted in the liver to ketones which act in the brain as an alternative fuel to glucose. Dr. Newport felt she was on to something.

When Steve tested the next morning, his score was too low, and he did not qualify for the clinical trial. Fortunately, he was scheduled for another screening test the next day.

On the trip home, Dr. Newport purchased coconut oil for Steve to try before the second screening test and hoped that he would score high enough to qualify for the trial. She found the composition of coconut oil on the USDA website and learned that it included nearly 60% MCT Oil. The night before, Dr. Newport learned that MCT Oil is partly converted in the liver to ketones which act as an alternative fuel to glucose in the brain. The next morning, she gave him a little over 2 ½ tbsp for his morning dose before heading to the hospital.

In the second test, he scored above the minimum score required for acceptance in the clinical trial. That same day Steve remembered the name of the city and the name of the hospital he was in and answered other questions Dr. Newport asked. They were both excited. When they returned home, Dr. Newport continued to give him coconut oil twice a day which includes MCT Oil and took the same amount herself. She would not give him something she was not willing to take herself.

After two weeks, Dr. Newport was happy to report that Steve had his life back. He could think more clearly, speak full sentences and smile again. He returned to his usual joking around when he woke up every morning. They could travel again.

Dr. Newport's first book was released in 2011, Alzheimer's Disease: What If There Was a Cure? The Story of Ketones. Her latest effort was released in August 2015 and is titled, The Coconut Oil and Low Carbohydrate Solution for Alzheimer's, Parkinson's and Other Diseases, A Guide to using Diet and a High-Energy Food to Protect and Nourish the Brain. You can access Dr. Newport's book here: coconutketones.com/alzheimers-book-store/

Dr. Newport recommends non-hydrogenated, virgin, organic coconut oil for best results. Non-hydrogenated contains no cholesterol and no trans-fat. She points out that many good coconut oils with MCT Oil can now be found on Amazon, Wal-

Mart, and in many mainstream grocery stores now. To start, Dr. Newport recommends a smaller dose of 1 tsp in the morning and evening to allow the digestive system to adjust and avoid diarrhea. Consult with your physician about your health before taking this or any product.

Strategy:

- After reading Steve's story, you are more knowledgeable about the benefits of Coconut Oil to help restore memory loss when taken daily. If you or a family member has been diagnosed with Alzheimer's or other dementia types, it can allow you to enjoy a better life while waiting for a cure to be found.

Suggestions:

- To provide ketones to the brain as an alternative fuel, take adequate amounts of Coconut Oil which includes MCT Oil daily.

Remember Dr. Newport's suggestion about starting with a smaller dose by taking 1 tsp in the morning and 1 tsp in the evening for two weeks. Increase to 2 1/2 tbsp twice daily to allow the digestive system to adjust and, avoid diarrhea.

For more information visit Dr. Mary Newport's website and blog:

- coconutketones.com
- coconutketones.blogspot.com

See Dr. Newport's nine-page detailed report
Coconut Oil: Dietary Guidelines and Suggestions **in the Appendix Section**

About the Lauric Acid in Coconut Oil & Ketone Salts

Lauric Acid in Coconut Oil

There is a new study out per the Journal of Oleo Sciences showing that lauric acid (half of the fat in coconut oil but usually a smaller amount in MCT Oil) increases ketone production in astrocytes which are brain cells that nourish the neurons...another good reason to keep coconut oil in the diet.

Ketone Salts Combined with MCT Oil

There is also a new product out that increases ketone levels much higher than coconut oil or MCT oil called **Pruvit,** ketone salts that contain the actual ketone betahydroxybutyrate and could bring about even more improvement; the orange flavor is combined with MCT. This could be part of the strategy, keeping coconut and MCT oil as the foundation. For elderly people or those with chronic medical conditions I recommend getting doctor's approval, so that electrolytes can be monitored and suggest starting slowly, – start with 1 or 2 level teaspoons of the ketone salts powder once or twice a day. Increase gradually over a week or two to 1/2 to 1 full serving daily. Some people decide to take more than one serving a day.

Also, very important - the person taking the salts needs to be able to drink plenty of fluids to avoid a dehydrating effect of raising ketones. [2]

References:

1. Newport, Dr., Mary (n.d.). Six video interviews/Steve's story. Retrieved April 2016 from CoconutKetones.com

2. Newport, Dr., M. (n.d.). Dr. Mary Newport's review of ketones and Pruvit. Retrieved March 31, 2017, from CoconutKetones.com

Photo Credits:

- Decanter with Coconut Oil and Coconuts – 37320955canstockphoto.ccom

CHAPTER 8

FOCUSED ULTRASOUND PROCEDURE

Non-Invasive Option to Get Your Life Back

It is exciting to locate promising dementia research. I read an intriguing report about Focused Ultrasound Procedure that is used to treat Parkinson's, Alzheimer's, and malignant and benign tumors. If you or a loved one experiences any of these symptoms, be sure to explore this non-invasive option to get your life back. Check out the *Clinical Trials* database link below.

Renowned author John Grisham and Dr. John Kassell, Chairman of the Focused Ultrasound Foundation (FUSF), spoke at TEDx in Charlottesville on November 13, 2015. They discussed the potential of using focused ultrasound to treat these medical conditions.

Grisham joined the FUSF Board of Directors six years ago after learning about the therapy's promise. His goal is to help raise awareness about the treatment.

Kimberly Spletter, the first person in the United States treated with focused ultrasound as part of the Michael J. Fox Foundation (MJFF) and FUSF-sponsored clinical trial was also on stage during the talk. "*My life before my focused ultrasound procedure was completely different*," said Spletter, who had great difficulty walking and could no longer complete some of her favorite activities like bike riding.

She stood strong on the stage and shared how she had walked back to her room immediately after the procedure. Kimberly wrote a short essay for the Michael J. Fox Foundation in September about her experience with the focused ultrasound treatment. Her essay is posted on the MJFF website at michaeljfox.org.

John Grisham has written another book. His newest piece of fiction, *The Tumor*, tells the story of a man diagnosed with a brain tumor and the opportunity that focused ultrasound affords his treatment. His book promotes focused ultrasound as a groundbreaking medical treatment.

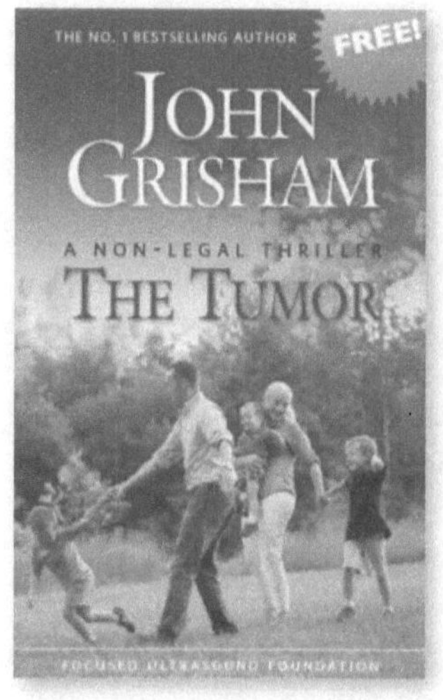

John Grisham had this to say,

"As a lawyer turned author, I know little about medicine and medical research. But when I learned about focused ultrasound and its potential to change lives, I knew it was a story worth telling. This is the most important book I have ever written. I have found no other cause that can potentially save so many lives. One day, in the not-too-distant future, you or someone you love will be diagnosed with a tumor. After the shock, you will think of focused ultrasound. Let's hope it's available."

Get your FREE e-book or hard copy from the Focused Ultrasound Foundation.

Brain Program

The Foundation considers the brain to be the vanguard target for focused ultrasound. Given the challenges of accessing the brain and the high cost, complications and limitations of some current approaches, we believe that this non-invasive technology has the potential to revolutionize the treatment of many brain disorders. It has the potential to:

- transform treatment by gaining access deep within the brain without harming healthy tissue;
- ablate targeted tissue without exposing the brain to the effects of ionizing radiation;
- enable the reversible opening of the blood-brain barrier to deliver therapeutic agents to targeted diseased areas;
- noninvasively dissolve blood clots that cause stroke; and
- noninvasively and reversibly modulate neural activity

It is the ultimate goal of the Foundation's Brain Program to see focused ultrasound become a standard of care for the treatment of a range of neurological disorders, including movement disorders, brain tumors, epilepsy and stroke.

The Foundation works with clinicians, researchers, and industry experts from around the world to identify critical challenges and design research to overcome them.

To date the Foundation has held six brain workshops that have succeeded in defining clear research objectives for clinical, preclinical and technical investigation.

Clinical studies have been launched investigating the treatment of movement disorders, including essential tremor and Parkinson's disease. The Foundation's technical research program involves a vibrant community of experts around the world to solve the challenges of applying focused ultrasound to an increasing array of high-impact, clinically unmet needs.

We are currently working with leading neurosurgery research centers to advance focused ultrasound for several movement disorders. The recent publication of focused ultrasound treatment for essential tremor in The New England Journal of Medicine is an incredible milestone for our Brain Program and demonstrates the potential of the technology. Based on this promising research, a clinical trial is starting in the U.S. that may lead to FDA approval of focused ultrasound for the treatment of essential tremor. Clinical research is also underway to study Parkinsonian tremor and dyskinesia.

We believe that focused ultrasound technology has the potential to make the practice of neurosurgery safer, faster, more effective and less costly.

Participating in Clinical Trials

Patient participation in clinical trials is critical to advancing focused ultrasound treatment for brain disorders. Research for essential tremor, Parkinsonian tremor and dyskinesia in Parkinson's disease is being planned or conducted with patients at a few leading centers. To find out more, you can search our clinical trials database.[1]

References:

1. The Focused Ultrasound Foundation (FUSF) (2013, November 1), Brain program. Retrieved from https://www.fusfoundation.org/for-researchers/high-priority-research-areas/brain-program

Photo Credits:

1. John Grisham – A Non-Legal Thriller – The Tumor. Retrieved from https://www.fusfoundation.org/read-the-tumor-by-john-grisham

CHAPTER 9

VITAMIN D DEFICIENCY LINKED TO DEMENTIA

There Are Three Ways to Get Vitamin D Levels Up to a Normal Level:

1. Get out of the house for a daily dose of sunshine

2. Eat foods with Vitamin D, such as oily fish, and,

3. Take Vitamin D supplements.

Trying to decrease your risk of dementia by eating more Vitamin D foods will be difficult, and you won't always be able to get a daily dose of sunshine.

Most likely, you need to include all three methods to ensure you are getting enough Vitamin D every day.

During my annual physical two years ago, the lab work showed a Vitamin D deficiency. The results surprised me because I have never had that problem. My doctor recommended taking 1000 to 2000 IU supplements daily.

I continue to take Vitamin D supplements but increased it to 4,000 IU per day to keep it at a normal level. I get Vitamin D from the fish I eat twice a week and try to get 15 minutes of sunshine daily as much as possible.

http://SandraPye.com/contact

There is a link between Alzheimer's and Vitamin D explained below. Keep your Vitamin D at a normal level to ensure you are taking the steps necessary to prevent the risk of dementia.

What Is the Link between Alzheimer's Disease and Vitamin D?

Researchers have found that there is a link between Vitamin D and the way the brain works. Researchers are beginning to study if not getting enough Vitamin D may affect whether you develop dementias, including AD.

Receptors for Vitamin D have been found in many parts of the brain. Receptors are found on the surface of a cell where they receive chemical signals. By attaching themselves to a receptor, these chemical signals direct a cell to do something; for example, to act in a certain way, or to divide or die.

Some of the receptors in the brain are receptors for Vitamin D, which means that Vitamin D is acting in some way in the brain and influencing the way an individual thinks, learns, and acts. Scientists have found that in people with AD, there are fewer Vitamin D receptors in a part of the brain called the hippocampus, which is involved in forming memories.

The brain relies on Vitamin D receptors for protection against the things that can damage it, including the development of the plaques and tangles that form in AD. How getting enough Vitamin D affects a brain with dementia is still being studied, but scientists do know that Vitamin D receptors work in many ways to protect the brain. However, these researchers are still exploring whether taking Vitamin D supplements can help prevent memory loss and dementia.[1]

How Do I Get the Vitamin D My Body Needs?

The two main ways to get Vitamin D are by exposing your bare skin to sunlight and by taking Vitamin D supplements. You can't get the right amount of Vitamin D your body needs from food.

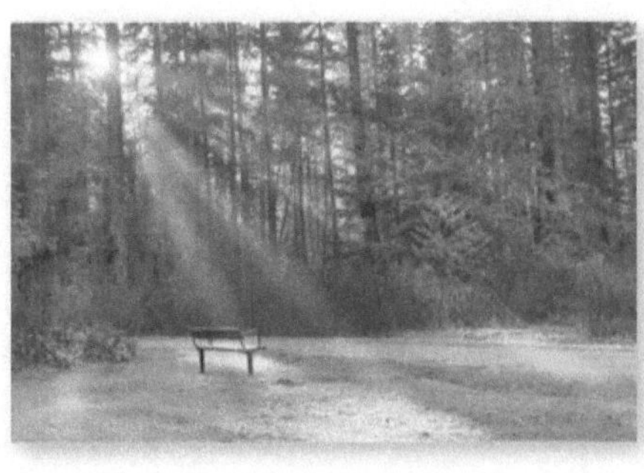

The most natural way to get Vitamin D is by exposing your bare skin to sunlight (ultraviolet B rays). This can happen very quickly, particularly in the summer. You don't need to tan or burn your skin to get Vitamin D. You only need to expose your skin for around half the time it takes for your skin to turn pink and begin to burn. How much Vitamin D is produced from sunlight depends on the time of day, where you live in the world and the color of your skin. The more skin you expose the more Vitamin D is produced.

You can also get Vitamin D by taking supplements. This is a good way to get Vitamin D if you can't get enough sunlight, or if you're worried about exposing your skin. Vitamin D3 is the best kind of supplement to take. It comes in a number of different forms, such as tablets and capsules, but it doesn't matter what form you take, or what time of the day you take it.

Different organizations recommend different amounts of Vitamin D supplement to take each day. The Vitamin D Council recommends taking larger amounts of Vitamin D each day than other organizations, because smaller amounts aren't enough to give you what your body needs. Most people can take Vitamin

D supplements with no problems. However, if you have certain health problems or take certain medicines, you may need to take extra care. [2]

You can now test your Vitamin D levels at home with an in-home Vitamin D Test Kit from Vitamin D Council's website.

References:

1. Vitamin D Council. (2015, November 30). What is the link between Alzheimer's and Vitamin D? Retrieved from https://www.Vitamindcouncil.org/health-conditions/alzheimers-disease/

2. The Vitamin D Council, About Vitamin D. https://www.Vitamindcouncil.org/about-Vitamin-d/ how-do-i-get-the-Vitamin-d-my-body-needs/

Photo Credits:

- Vitamin D pill – 28008584canstockphoto.com
- Green Park with Bench / Sunshine – 33100111canstockphoto.com

SECTION V

Conclusion

CHAPTER 10

THE CONCLUSION

Things I Could Do to Prevent Dementia

I have spent many hours on research. The driving force of this passionate endeavor was to avoid getting caught in the grips of a downward spiral of dementia. I did not want to one day find myself in the middle of a slow decline in memory and cognitive abilities like my mother experienced.

My goal was to learn as much as possible to create a plan of action to prevent or reduce my risk of dementia. As I continued my research, I decided that I wanted to organize all my notes into a book that may help other people.

Age-Related 'Normal' Occasional "Senior Moments"

The phrase, *senior moments,* is a common term that is used to describe senior citizens. So, I accepted it when Mother experienced occasional moments of memory loss. An adult person, who is not even 55 years of age, can experience normal or occasional age-related senior moments and pass them off as *normal* and *expected.* It can even conjure up shared giggles when a person says, "Oops, excuse me, I'm having a senior moment."

There may come a time when a person fails to grasp that senior moments are coming around too often to be normal and that their thinking skills are slowing and not up to par. The sooner a person or family member recognizes this and takes action, the better off they will be.

http://SandraPye.com/contact

Get Very Serious about Reversing The Downward Spiral

My research provided much better insight about what I could have done to help Mother avoid dementia. I should have been more aware when her normal and occasional "senior moments" increased into too many senior moments with confusion.

When This Is Happening, It's Time To Come Up with A Plan

Be alert if this happens to you or a loved one and come up with a plan to prevent further decline in memory and thinking skills. Accept the possibility it could be the start of a more serious problem such as Mild Cognitive Impairment (MCI).

Mild Cognitive Impairment (MCI)

With "amnestic MCI" there are memory problems where a person may forget appointments, conversations, and recent events.

With "non-amnestic MCI" a person will experience a decline in thinking skills other than memory, including the ability to make sound decisions or judge time.

IMPORTANT: A person with MCI is at an increased risk of developing Alzheimer's disease or another type of dementia.

Revisit Chapter 1, Mild Cognitive Impairment (MCI) to review this information.

BE ALERT! The chart below is a helpful reminder to stay alert to prevent the spiraling effect of dementia for you, your family and friends. If you have not seen the devastating effects of dementia or felt the sadness and pain that goes with it, you are fortunate.

You may view this chart as a curiosity. If so, quell that curiosity and learn what you can do today to keep your brain healthy and alert.

However, you wouldn't be reading this book if you weren't curious, right? Congratulations about being pro-active about your brain health.

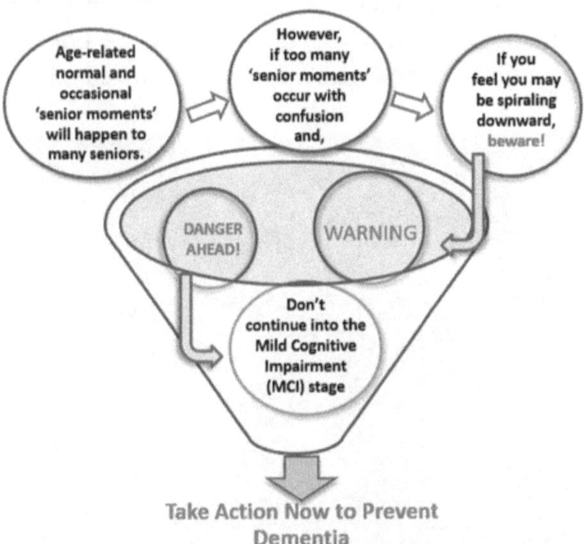

1. DIET: Eat healthy – eat more brain food, eat less junk food.
2. PHYSICAL ACTIVITY: Exercise regularly – walking, cycling or, other activities.
3. MENTAL ACTIVITY: Be consistent with mental stimulation. Learn new skills, play board games, word search or crossword puzzles.
4. WELLNESS: Get a good night's sleep, don't smoke, and, control high blood pressure.

http://SandraPye.com/contact

This sad experience drove me to learn everything I could about dementia and fed the need deep in my heart and soul to share what I learned.

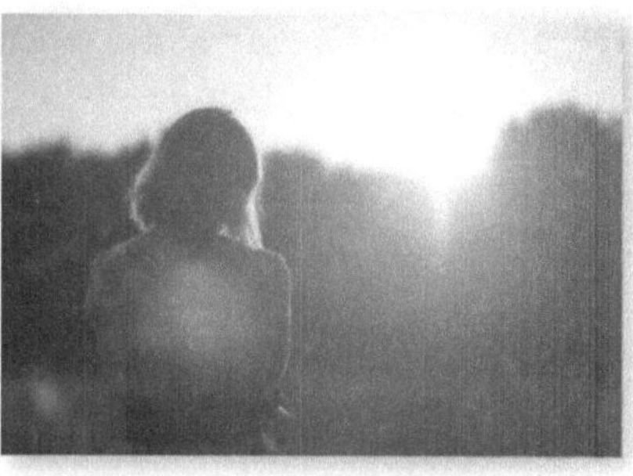

By sharing my thoughts, tips and suggestions, sweet and sad memories, and research information, I hope you find this simple book a helpful guide for you or a loved one.

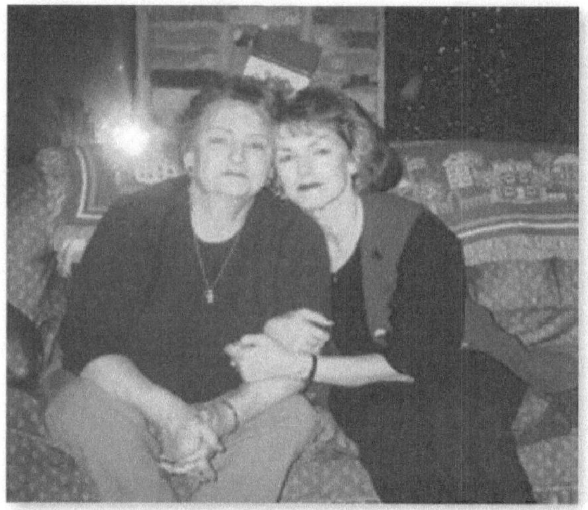

*Mother and I sharing sweet and precious time
together on Christmas Eve-pre-dementia*

APPENDIX

COCONUT OIL DIETARY GUIDELINES SUGGESTIONS

Report published with permission from Dr. Mary T. Newport, MD.
See CoconutKetones.com for more information

How Can Coconut Oil Be Used in the Diet?

Coconut oil can be substituted for any solid or liquid oil, lard, butter, or margarine in baking or cooking on the stove, and can be mixed directly into foods already prepared. Some people take it straight with a spoon, but for most people it may be hard to swallow this way and more pleasant to take with food.

When cooking on the stove, coconut oil smokes if heated to greater than 350 degrees or medium heat. You can avoid this problem by adding a little olive or peanut oil. Coconut oil can be used at any temperature in the oven when mixed in foods.

What Is the Nutrient Content of Coconut Oil? Does It Contain Omega-3 Fatty Acids?

Coconut oil has about 117-120 calories per tablespoon, about the same as other oils. It contains 57-60% medium chain triglycerides (MCT), which are absorbed directly without the need for digestive enzymes. Part of it is metabolized by the liver to ketones which can be used by most cells in the body for energy. This portion of the coconut oil is not stored as fat.

Coconut oil is about 86% saturated fat, most of which is the medium chain fats that are metabolized differently than animal saturated fats. It contains no cholesterol and no trans-fat, as long as is non-hydrogenated. An advantage of a saturated fat is that there is nowhere on the molecule for free radicals or oxidants to attach.

About 6% of the oil is monounsaturated and 2% polyunsaturated. Coconut oil also contains a small amount of phytosterols, which are one of the components of the "statins" used for lowering cholesterol.

Coconut oil contains omega-6 fatty acids but **no omega-3 fatty acid**, so this must be taken in addition to coconut oil. You can obtain all of the essential fatty acids required by using just coconut oil and omega-3 fatty acids. If you were to use coconut oil as your primary oil, the only other oil you would need is an omega-3 fatty acid, which you can get by eating salmon twice a week, or taking fish oil or flax oil capsules, 2-3 per day. Some other good sources of omega-3 fatty acids are ground flax meal, chia (a fine grain), walnut oil and walnuts.

Lauric acid is a medium chain triglyceride that makes up almost half of the coconut oil. Scientific studies show that lauric acid has antimicrobial properties and may inhibit growth of certain bacteria, fungus/yeast, viruses and protozoa. It is one of the components of human breast milk that prevents infection in a newborn.

What Kind of Coconut Oil Should I Use?

Look for coconut oils that are non-hydrogenated with no trans-fat. Avoid coconut oils that are hydrogenated or superheated because it changes the chemical structure of the fats.

If you like the odor of coconut, look for products called "virgin," "organic," or "unrefined," which are generally more expensive than "refined," or "all natural," or "RBD" (refined, bleached and deodorized) coconut oil, which do not have an odor. The oil itself is tasteless. Any of these have essentially the same nutrient with about 57-60% MCT oil (medium chain triglycerides).

The least expensive that I have been able to find so far is the Louana brand at Walmart, priced locally at $5.44 per quart. Using **coconut oil capsules is not an efficient way** to give the oil since the capsules are relatively expensive and contain only 1 gram of oil per capsule, whereas the oil is 14 grams per tablespoon. Capsules might be useful for someone who will not take the oil.

Why Does the Coconut Oil Look "Cloudy"?

Coconut oil is a clear or slightly yellow liquid above 76 degrees but becomes solid at 76 degrees and below. If your house is kept right around 76 degrees you may even see partly liquid oil with solid clouds of oil floating in it. If your home is generally kept at 75 degrees or below, the oil will tend to be a white or slightly yellow soft semi-solid.

What Other Coconut Products Contain Coconut Oil?

Coconut milk is a combination of the oil and the water from the coconut and most of the calories are from the oil. Look for brands with 10 to 13 grams of fat in 2 ounces. Look in the grocery store's Asian section. Some brands are less expensive but are diluted with water. **Coconut cream** is mostly coconut milk and sometimes has added sugar.

Flaked or grated coconut can be purchase unsweetened or sweetened and is a very good source of coconut oil and fiber and has about 15 grams oil and 3 grams fiber in ¼ cup. Frozen or canned **coconut meat** usually has a lot of added sugar and not much oil per serving. A **fresh coconut** can be cut up into pieces and eaten raw. A 2" x 2" piece has about 160 calories with 15 grams of oil and 4 grams of fiber.

MCT Oil (medium chain triglycerides) are part of the coconut oil and can also be purchased in some health food stores or on-line. This may be useful for people who are on the go and do not have much time to cook. Also, MCT oil is used as energy and not stored as fat, so it may be useful for someone who wants to lose weight, if substituted for some of the other fats in the diet.

Coconut water does not usually contain coconut oil, but has other health benefits. The electrolyte composition is similar to human plasma and is useful to prevent or treat dehydration.

How Should I Store Coconut Products?

Coconut oil is extremely stable with a shelf life of at least two years when stored at room temperature. It does not need to be refrigerated and becomes extremely hard when cold.

If you wish to keep it in the refrigerator, you can measure out 1 or 2 tablespoons into each section of a plastic ice cube tray. The coconut oil easily pops out of the plastic tray.

Coconut milk is mostly coconut oil and can be substituted for the oil in many ways. Coconut milk must be refrigerated after opening and should be used within a few days or tossed out. Grated or flaked coconut can be stored at room temperature for a few weeks, but may last longer if stored in a refrigerator. A freshly cut up coconut can be stored in the refrigerator for a few days or freezer for a couple of weeks.

Who Should Try This?

People who have a neurodegenerative disease that involves decreased glucose uptake in neurons could benefit from taking higher amounts of coconut and/or MCT oil to produce ketones which may be used by brain cells as energy. These diseases include Alzheimer's and other dementias, Parkinson's, ALS (Lou Gehrig's), multiple sclerosis (MS), Duchenne muscular dystrophy, autism, Down's syndrome, and Huntington's chorea.

Ketones can also serve as an alternative fuel for other cells in the body that are insulin resistant or cannot transport glucose, and could potentially lessen the effects of diabetes I or II on the brain and other organs.

If you are at risk due to family history, you consider making this dietary change as well. If your loved one is in assisted living, the doctor may be willing to prescribe coconut oil to be given at each meal, increasing gradually.

How Much Should I Take?

If you take too much oil too fast, you may experience indigestion, cramping or diarrhea. To avoid these symptoms, take with food and start with 1 teaspoon coconut oil or MCT oil per meal, increasing slowly as tolerated over a week or longer. If diarrhea develops, drop back to the previous level.

For most people, the goal would be to increase gradually to 4-6 tablespoons a day, depending on the size of the person, spread over 2-4 meals.

Mixing MCT oil and coconut oil could provide higher levels and a steady level of ketones. One formula is to mix 16 ounces MCT oil plus 12 ounces coconut oil in a quart jar and increase slowly as tolerated, starting with 1 teaspoon. This mixture will stay liquid at room temperature.

What about Children?

Children with Down's syndrome and some children with autism show decreased glucose uptake in parts of the brain. A reasonable amount to give a child would be about ¼ teaspoon of coconut oil for every 10 pounds that the child weighs 2 or 3 times a day.

Also, some children like the taste of coconut milk - 1½ to 2 teaspoons per 10 pounds weight can be added to the diet 2 or 3 times a day. If you use coconut milk for a child, be sure to refrigerate it and discard after two days. Do not add honey to coconut milk for children under 1 year old, due to risk of infection.

Do I Need to Be Worried about Gaining Weight from the Extra Fat in the Diet?

Yes!! The best way to avoid gaining weight is to <u>substitute</u> coconut oil for most other fats and oils in the diet, and if that isn't enough, cut back on portion sizes of carbohydrates, such as breads, rice, potatoes, cereals, and other grains.

In general it is a good idea to use whole milk products but, if weight gain is a problem, you can also compensate for some of the new fat in the diet by changing from full fat to lower fat dairy products, such as milk, cheese, cottage cheese and yogurts, as well as low-fat or fat-free salad dressings, to which you can add coconut oil.

Also, use a measuring spoon and remove the excess by leveling it with a knife to avoid overestimating, which can make a big difference in the number of calories consumed.

Tiny glass measuring cups are available at grocery stores with markings for teaspoons and tablespoons. These are especially useful for combining salad dressing with coconut oil.

Does Coconut Oil Increase Cholesterol?

<u>Hydrogenated</u> coconut oil can increase cholesterol. Therefore, look for <u>non</u>-hydrogenated coconut oil with no trans-fat There is no cholesterol in coconut oil itself, and with *nonhydrogenated* coconut oil, most people will see little difference or will see an improvement in their HDL ("good") and a decrease in LDL ("bad") cholesterol.

Some see an increase in total cholesterol, usually as a result of an increase in HDL ("good") cholesterol.

Some Other Benefits of Coconut Oil and Other Coconut Products

Coconut oil is easily absorbed by the body and increases absorption of certain vitamins and minerals and other important nutrients. This would also hold true for coconut milk, coconut meat, whether wet or dry, such as flaked or grated coconut.

The fiber in coconut meat may be especially beneficial to persons with Crohn's or other types of inflammatory bowel disease or malabsorption syndromes and people who have diarrhea from MCT or coconut oil.

All of your cell membranes and about 60-70% of the brain and are made up of fats. Cholesterol is a very important component of the support structure of the brain. Many cell functions take place within the cell membrane. Since about the 1950's many people in this country have been using 100% vegetable oil, which is usually hydrogenated polyunsaturated fat and contains trans-fat, which can carry free radicals into your cell membranes.

If you begin to substitute coconut and other natural oils, such as olive oil and even butter, along with omega-3 oils you may be able to undo some of the damage. Most of the cells of the body turn over within 3 to 6 months and you may notice a nicer texture to your skin, and a decrease in certain problems such as yeast and fungal infections.

Food Ideas

- Use coconut oil instead of butter on toast, English muffins, bagels, grits, corn on the cob, potatoes, sweet potatoes, rice, vegetables, noodles, pasta.
- Mix coconut oil into oatmeal or other hot cereal.
- Add coconut oil or milk to smoothies, yogurt or kefir.
- Mix coconut oil half and half with salad dressings.
- Mix coconut oil into your favorite soup, chili or sauce.
- Use a measured amount of coconut oil to stir fry or sauté (add peanut oil over medium heat)
- Purchase or make coconut macaroons made from all natural products.
- Eat a 2" x 2" square of raw coconut for a snack to provide 15 grams of oil.
- Add flaked or grated coconut to hot or cold cereal, yogurt, fruit or vegetable salads.
- "The Coconut Lover's Cookbook," Bruce Fife – many more great ideas

Recipes

Coconut Macaroons:

- 2 egg whites   Dash of salt
  1/2 tsp vanilla
- 2/3 cup sugar or 1/4 cup sugar and 1 to 2 dashes of Stevia extract
- 1 cup shredded coconut

Beat egg whites with salt and vanilla until soft peaks form. Gradually add sugar (and Stevia), beating until stiff. Fold in coconut. Coat cooking sheet with generous amount of butter. Drop by the rounded teaspoon onto cookie sheet. Bake at 325 degrees for 20 minutes. Makes about 18 cookies. Each cookie at this size would have about 4 grams of coconut oil.

Coconut Milk:

- Mix in a container and shake well before use:
- can of coconut milk ½ can of water Dash of salt
- 1-2 tablespoons of honey or another sweetener to taste

Store in refrigerator and discard unused portion after 4 days.

"Fudge"

Melt and mix together **1 cup each** of coconut oil and chocolate chips and divide equally into a plastic ice cube tray and place in freezer. In a 16 cube tray, each cube will equal 1 tablespoon coconut oil. Add grated coconut and/or nuts for variety.

MCT Oil/Coconut Oil Mixture

Store at room temperature, in a quart size jar:

- 16 ounces MCT oil + 12 ounces coconut oil

www.ingramcontent.com/pod-product-compliance
Lightning Source LLC
Chambersburg PA
CBHW051104250726

48656CB00001B/463